Plyometrics and Vertical Jump

How to Increase Your Vertical Jump

(Increase Your Vertical Jump in Volleyball and Basketball)

Stephen Carter

Published By **Oliver Leish**

Stephen Carter

Plyometrics and Vertical Jump: How to Increase Your Vertical Jump (Increase Your Vertical Jump in Volleyball and Basketball)

ISBN   978-1-77485-965-0

No part of this guidebook shall be reproduced in any form without permission in writing from the publisher except in the case of brief quotations embodied in critical articles or reviews.

Legal & Disclaimer

Upon using the information contained in this book, you agree to hold harmless the Author from and against any damages, costs, and expenses, including any legal fees potentially resulting from the application of any of the information provided by this guide. This disclaimer applies to any damages or injury caused by the use and application, whether directly or indirectly, of any advice or information presented, whether for breach of contract, tort, negligence, personal injury, criminal intent, or under any other cause of action.

You agree to accept all risks of using the information presented inside this book. You need to consult a professional medical practitioner in order to ensure you are both able and healthy enough to participate in this program.

Table of contents

Chapter 1: The value of dunking

The dunk, one of the most iconic moves in basketball, is undoubtedly synonymous with it. This high-flying move makes basketball so special. It is more than a trademark shot. It is one of most remarkable feats athleticism in all sports. It's not easy, so it isn't for everyone. The basketball slamdunk has real value beyond its glamour. Here are some of the reasons why slam dunk in basketball is important, especially for those who can do it.

1. It's a high percentage shot. Because the ball is literally slammed into the rim, it's the most accurate shot in basketball. You can almost guarantee success with the slam dunk. This is why the catchphrase was created. Dunking is so deadly, in fact, that it was banned in basketball for giving some teams and players an unfair advantage. Dunking is not only a beautiful skill, but it's also a vital skill that should be part of any

basketball game plan. If you are able to execute it properly, you won't miss a dunk.

2. It is a great way for you to build your confidence. You can say it like a basketball quote: "It only takes the ball to go through the basket for it to start." You don't have to win the entire game, it doesn't matter how hard it is. Just get one shot in and it might change your mood. A slam dunk can change the mood. You can feel confident when you are able to get up for a jam. Not only will you feel confident, but your team could also feel that way. A successful dunk will boost your team's morale, and it can even change the game's momentum in your favor.

3. It is a high-quality entertainment activity. The slam doug is a crowd-pleasing staple. A successful dunk will always be a great way to get people moving during games. The dunk is an extraordinary feat of athleticism. It combines power, athleticism, and grace into one powerful move. However, a dunk may take many forms and occur at times

when you least expect them. The moment a player does a spectacular dunk in shootaround or during a playoff match, everyone is amazed and applauds it. The bottom line, the slam dance has incredible entertainment value.

4. It will increase your chances of getting noticed. Teams assess talent based upon a number of criteria. Athleticism is one important parameter. Jumping ability is an important aspect of athleticism that is often considered by teams. People who can jump high above their opponents have an advantage on the court. Dunking the basket is a great way of demonstrating your athletic ability, especially for those who are below-average or average height. Basketball scouts look for potential. And nothing speaks more of potential than a huge slam, dunk.

5. Your ability to dunk tells a lot of things about your athletic abilities. As was mentioned before, the best feats for

athleticism in any sport is dunking. It is easy to see why. It takes athletic ability and skill to be able or capable of dunk. Basketball today is all about athleticism, and the ability of a dunk is a great demonstration.

Basketball is not complete without dunk. You don't necessarily have to be able to dunk to be a good basketball player. However, having it in your arsenal is an excellent asset. The good news is that even though you may not be a naturally-born dunker, it doesn't have to be that way. You can learn dunking regardless of your height or gender. The next pages will teach you how to fly and make dunks.

Chapter 2: Developing your Vertical Jump

There are many factors which can impact your chances of landing a slam shot. People would assume that height is the main factor. But, it was again disproved time and time again by basketball players who are below 6 feet. Their ability to jump is the greatest factor that divides dunkers from non-dunkers. The first step to becoming a slam ducker is to improve your vertical jump. Your leap can be made more explosive and inches taller with proper training. These are some tips to increase your vertical jump.

1. Get rid of excess weight. Your vertical jump won't increase if you are carrying too much weight. This is just the law of physics. If your weight doesn't allow you to jump higher, it will make you jump lower. You'll need extra weight to lift your legs. To do this, you should get leaner. Cardio exercise and high intensity interval training are two ways to lose fat. Your excess weight can be reduced by managing your food intake and

habits. You can achieve your ideal weight by combining regular exercise with healthy eating habits.

2. Use deadlifts and squats. Two of the most basic exercise routines are the deadlift or squat. This is a set of exercises that strengthens your whole body. Deadlifts and squats target the quadriceps and hamstrings muscle groups, which generate most of your legs' upward force. This exercise also helps to strengthen your core and back for jumping. You should do at least 10 reps of each set and use a weight that is sufficiently challenging for you to be successful in both.

3. Do calf raises. Calf muscles are essential for jumping mechanics. Studies have shown that quads and the hamstrings are less important in determining jump power. However, powering your calves will improve your vertical jump. The effective extension of your ankles can help make the contractions of your hips, thigh and thigh muscles easier. Calf raises work the best to

target the calves. It can either be done using your body weight or with additional resistance. You can also perform the exercise in sets, or as an endurance challenge.

4. Flexibility can help you achieve greater success. Flexibility is crucial if you want higher jumps. It goes like this: The more flexible your muscles become, the more you are able to contract with greater force. It also balances the forces generated within your body. Flexibility and extension of your legs allows you to maximize momentum. This leads to stronger and more powerful leaps. Good stretching helps reduce muscle injuries during games or training. After working out, make sure you stretch your buttocks. You'll find that flexibility improves with regular stretching.

5. Plyometrics. This is one the most used catch phrases in the field of athletic training. Plyometric exercise uses your body's resistance to build strength and

explosiveness. The goal of plyometric exercise is to make your muscles contract at maximum force in a short time. This allows you make fast, explosive jumps which are important for many basketball skills other than dunking. Plyometrics can improve your jumping ability and speed, as well. This set of exercises should be done regularly.

6. Jumping drills. Jumping practice is crucial for many reasons. Jumping practice is a great way of strengthening your muscles and increasing your vertical leap. It also teaches you how and when to jump correctly. This will increase your elevation. It also helps you balance and improve your footwork. These are essential for performing the quick, controlled moves required to play basketball. Fourth, it increases your coordination, stamina, and is necessary for performing second and subsequent jumps in quick succession. Jumping drills that are effective include box drills, squat jumps, and backboard touches.

Your jump will take time. You can be confident that there are many ways to get the results that you desire. Use all these techniques to improve your vertical jump. These drills could help you turn that slam into a slam.

Chapter 3: Improve Your Jumping Technique

The last chapter addressed the subtleties of increasing your jump by increasing fitness and strengthening the muscles that are used to jump. Although power is essential, it is not the only factor that will allow you to achieve maximum elevation. In order to maximize the power flowing to your legs, you must improve your jumping technique. Good jumping technique improves the efficiency of every movement, ensuring that vertical propulsion is achieved with every ounce of power your body produces. Here are the steps to improving your jumping technique.

1. It is important to practice jumping when you're at a standstill. It is crucial that you can still jump at full speed, or even half speed. This skill can be used to grab rebounds, block shots, collect putbacks, and even catch the ball. You need to ensure your feet touch the ground with both your feet.

By extending your knees slightly, you can force your body upwards. When your knees are straighten, extend your ankles. Your body should now be lifted off of the ground. Avoid any serious injuries by jumping with your body stabilized.

2. Try running while jumping. People are much more likely to dunk when they run. This is because forward momentum can increase the distance and height one can jump. It is crucial to be able jump with both one or two feet. Practice jumping while walking, jogging or running to improve your coordination. The jump should be smooth and coordinated. After mastering the jumping motion, practice running while jumping. Eventually, you will be able to run while jumping. Jump as if you were trying to do a dunk. It will help you improve your coordination as well as your confidence.

3. Learn how to land correctly. Every high-flying sport has inherent dangers. The same goes for dunks. Many players have been

seriously injured by being unable to properly land after a dunk attempt. It is important for every dunker to learn how safely to land. To land safely, especially after performing a full-force leap, such as the dunk attempt, you should land on both of your legs. Then, bend your knees slightly and flex your ankles to absorb any impact. If you have to land on one foot, or if landing on the other is impossible due to a running start, then make sure your landing transition is smooth as your legs touch the ground. Even before you take off, imagine how you'll land. If you don't feel confident about your landing, don't attempt to jump. While you will always have many opportunities to connect on your leap, you can't afford to lose them if it causes you unnecessary injury.

4. The ball is not required to go over the rim. Practice your hops with your ball in your hand later. The first thing you should learn is how to move above the rim. As your

body becomes more flexible and your strides are smoother, it will become easier and easier to get closer the rim. Your hands will soon reach the rim. In fact, you might end up way above the rim with a few attempts. Here, you will be learning proper leaping skills while also putting yourself in a position where the ball can be flushed to the rim. Once you are able to coordinate and time your movements correctly, you can begin dunk-training.

Your leaping ability is an essential step towards converting a slam to a basket. You need to be able to leap high enough for that slam. The next chapter will teach you everything you need to do to put the ball in the basket.

Chapter 4: Learn to Dunk

People rarely dunk their first attempt in games. Except for mitigating conditions, it's very rare that people convert their first slam attempt in games. Nearly all dunkers learned how to dunk at the gym while practicing basketball. Training is where ballers learn to safely and correctly dunk. This chapter will cover proper dunking techniques so you're ready to go when the opportunity arises during the game.

1. Learn how to control and move the ball. It is important to control the ball when you are throwing. For maximum effort when jumping towards the rim you must have complete control of the ball. Lack of ball control can impede momentum and make it easier to let your opponents steal your ball. Learn how to control your ball and improve your dribbling skills. When taking off, ensure that you hold the ball steadily using one or two fingers. This will make it easy to guide

the ball to its destination for the dunk. Through practice, ball control can be taught.

2. Practice dunking mechanics. Practice your dunking techniques with smaller equipment. If you want to feel like you are actually jumping with the ball, it is a good idea to start by dunking with smaller balls. This helps you learn important skills such as timing and elevation. If you are unable to master all of these with smaller balls, then you will not be able the standard basketball. Start with a tennis court. Once you feel you have the skills, you can use a tennis ball or a mini-basketball. Finally, you will practice dunking with a standard-sized basketball. This step is optional. You can also practice dunk at a shorter distance (you'll need an adjustable basketball for this purpose) before you move on to the 10-foot rim.

3. Learn effective body control. You must learn to control your body if you wish to become a good dunker. There is no legitimate slam dunker that looked

uncomfortable while flying towards or near the rim. It is vital to maintain body control for several reasons. First, it helps to avoid injuries from bad landings or takeoffs. It allows you make coordinated attacks to the rim. You can even make adjustments in midair if necessary. It aids in absorbing contact, evading defenders and creating beautiful facial dunks. With proper dunking form combined with physical strength, you can control your body.

4. Focus. Focus. Before you go off, this mindset is essential: get the ball in the basket! You must believe that you are able to go beyond the rim and conquer any challenge along the way. You have to believe in your ability to dunk. You can become the best dunker you can by having self-belief.

5. Be persistent. Newbies will be confronted with many challenges. There will be times where you don't hit the dunks. It could be during practice or during a match, and you

will miss the dunk. It is crucial that you don't make these mistakes but still continue to dunk. This is where you will learn and improve as a dunker. Continue practicing, and you'll be making rim-rattling Slams in no time.

Even for athletes with exceptional athleticism and talent, learning to dunk takes patience and practice. Follow the tips and you will soon master the slamdunk, even if your athleticism is not.

Chapter 5: Effective Techniques To Help You Get Started in Games

There is a big difference between being able and being able dunk during games. Every basketball player knows that it is much harder to perform any skill during a real game than in practice. Your ability to dunk is not the same as your ability to do it in practice. This chapter will help guide you as you transition from being "a dunker" to "a dunker in games".

1. Use everything you've learned in training. Everything you learned about dunking matters. It would be ineffective if it wasn't going to be used on the court. It is essential that you apply every technique that you learn during practice, from proper gathering before takeoff and landing after converting to a dunk. This would ensure that you are safe and a successful conversion.

2. Learn how you can pace yourself. It is vital to have the right energy levels when playing dunking. It is common for your body

to be less strong when you are tired. When you're tired, your body is less capable of giving you the lift you need. Therefore, to keep dunkin', you need to learn how energy can be conserved. This can be done by having the proper foundations. Your legs will be healthier if you do a simpler dunk. If you don't feel energetic enough to do the dunk it's fine. You can always do a layup.

3. Improve your stamina. Basketball is a physically demanding sport. You'll be constantly running and banging heads with other players. This can become exhausting and can affect your performance. You may find it hard to execute the majority of basketball plays or perform high-energy maneuvers like the dunking. This problem can be solved by proper game management and improving your stamina. Cardio training (running, cycling, and surprise, basketball) can increase your stamina so that you can stay longer on the courts.

4. Increase your physical strength. You don't have to be a high flyer to become a competent dunker. It is important to have good overall strength. Did you ever wonder how the best players can leap over defenders for facials. In addition to being able jump higher than opponents, they are also strong enough to absorb contact and still convert the ball. Strengthening your entire body through resistance training is a great way to do this. Your strength can be used by pushing yourself to the basket. By strengthening your skills, you can significantly increase your chances of winning at dunking.

5. Increase your mental toughness. As a basketball player, you need mental toughness. As a basketball player there are many methods to improve your mental toughness. Two key elements are your mental preparation prior to the game and your focus. Half of the mental battle is won if your mind and resolve are clear. If you

believe you can do anything, it will give you the confidence you need to try. Most importantly, being able to believe that you can do it would allow you to succeed on the court.

Individuals may have different difficulties when making the transition to being a game dunker from practice. For some, it may be easy. Others may need some adjustments. Once you master these, it will be easy to start slamdunking on the basketball court regularly. It's a matter if you are willing to work hard and it is possible.

Chapter 6: The Most Important Tips for Dunkers Everywhere

I am assuming that you are interested in learning how to dunk. These tips could prove to be very helpful as you begin to master the art of converting slam shots. These tips can be useful even for those who are not slam dunkers. Here are some tips I can offer to dunkers around the world.

1. Continue to work hard. Dunking is possible only by hard work. It's hard work that will enable you to keep dunking. While you may be able to do more than the others, it is not a good idea. You will lose your athletic ability if it isn't hard work to keep yourself prepared for the games. You will also lose your ability for slamdunks. You will need to continue working hard to improve your ability to dunk.

2. You should also learn other basketball skills. Other than slam dunk specialists, you should also learn other basketball skills. While you might be able and able to hit the

rim, your skills on the court will not be enough. Expand your game to increase your chances for more playing time. You can improve shooting, rebounding, defensive skills and become a more complete athlete. You can also learn how to play the particular position you are playing on the court. Not only are you a better dunker, but also you need to improve your game.

3. You can increase your basketball IQ. A player's basketball IQ can be defined as their knowledge and experience with the game. A player with high basketball intelligence is capable of making the right moves at exactly the right time. They can also maximize their athletic skills and abilities to make a difference in the team's success and win. Although some people may be born with a high basketball IQ, this does not necessarily mean that they are incapable of developing theirs. It is important to take the time to learn how to make good basketball plays. Make the most

of your individual skills to help your team win. It is important to be at the right location at the correct time. Basketball intelligence tends to increase with experience and intuition.

4. Don't do fancy dunks, unless you can actually do them right. Basketball is supposed be fun. Basketball is not supposed to be entertaining. It can actually be quite disgraceful when played in the wrong way. The slamdunk is one aspect of the game that's almost always popular. If you feel confident enough to perform the slam dunk, you can go ahead. Save it for the next day and go to the gym to perfect your showtime dunk. There are only a few things that basketball is more embarrassing than showboating. Remember what coaches have to say about showboating: It's still equivalent to 2 points. However, most situations will be fine with a simple dunk and layup.

5. Safety first A dunk is an airborne maneuver that can pose risks. When you go for a dunk, there are many ways to injure yourself or others. The first is to make sure the surface and your shoes don't get too slippery. It can be dangerous to slip at full speed. Do not hold onto the rim unless it is in danger of you hitting someone, or if your momentum is needed to make a safe landing. Third, you should check that the rim is stable enough to be able to dunk on. Do not attempt to dunk if you fear the rim might break or the backboard may collapse.

Chapter 7: Why Increase Your Vertical Jump

Why are people so obsessed with their vertical leaps? You want to be able jump higher to excel in your chosen sport. Consider basketball. It is possible to shoot the ball in the middle of the court or beyond the three points arc. However, your success rate at making a basket is lower than making a lay up or dunk. Your body must have the ability to produce explosive power that propels your body upwards.

Does your genetics matter?

"White men can't leap" is a myth that has been around for a long time. It is one of the most widespread misconceptions about how high a person can jump. Today, virtually everyone can leap gracefully into the air when they watch the NBA, or any other basketball match, and it is possible to remain there for an unbelievable amount of times.

It is true that you can reach higher heights if you are taller than others, but this doesn't mean you will be able to jump higher vertically if you're shorter. The more you leap, the more weight you must propel up. Your hands can reach higher than your feet, but your jump height will not increase as much. However, if your height is smaller than you think, you might be able to jump higher even though you have trained yourself to do so.

What types of sports require exceptional leaping ability

Although it is likely that your motivation for improving your vertical leaping ability was to play better in basketball, there are many sports where having great jumping abilities can help you get an edge.

Track-and-field

If you are interested in sprinting and other track sports, it might seem like increasing your vertical leaping ability is irrelevant. However, you will be shocked at how important it can be. If your legs can jump high, it means that your legs have the power to lift your body weight to a substantial height. This will give you the ability to take control of the start box and make a big impression.

Volleyball

For you to be able jump over the net and get the ball into the opponents' courts, as well as defend against their attacks, you must have exceptional jumping ability. Due to the fact that volleyball requires you to jump almost for the entire game, your stamina will be greatly improved if you train to increase your vertical leaping ability. You'll be able to play an entire match with no fatigue.

Rugby and Football

This explosive energy allows you to lift your body up, which is useful for full contact sports like rugby or football. For you to maneuver between defenders and sprint at speed, you'll need to have incredible leg strength. All of these activities require the same muscles as your vertical leap.

Vertical jumps can be achieved with the right training. This book will show you the various training techniques you can use to increase your legs' explosive energy and make it possible to leap to heights previously thought impossible.

Chapter 8: Vertical Jump Basics

Before you can improve vertical leaping abilities, you have to assess your current vertical leap. You will learn how accurately to measure your jumps in this chapter so you can see how your training has affected your ability.

What is the Vertical Jump?

Most people believe vertical jumping ability to be the height at which they can jump. Vertical jumping ability is measured in the height to which the person can jump off the ground. Do not confuse this with people who tuck their legs when they jump. This does not indicate that you can jump higher; it simply means you have a longer "hangtime".

A person 6'11" tall can dunk the basketball. It will appear that he only took a short hop to get to the ring. But, what if someone 5'11 is able to dunk the basketball? That is an amazing feat. Both of these players were capable of dunking the basketball. But the shorter player showed impressive jumping skills.

How to measure your current vertical jump

Here's an easy method to gauge your leaping ability. You will need some chalk, some measuring tape, comfortable sneakers, and non-constricting clothing. The first step is to crush some chalk, dip your fingers in the chalk dust, and then stand in front of the wall. This will mark the height at which you can jump.

Now, move backwards toward the wall. Then jump as high you can. Make sure to mark the highest point you can reach with chalk dust covered hands. You can measure the distance from your mark just standing up to the one left when you jumped to determine your current vertical jump.

It can be difficult for you to find numbers to compare your vertical leaping ability with. You need to consider body mass and height as well as core strength. For men between 21-35 years old and with a BMI 25 or higher, the average jump height is between 22-25 inches. Women can leap between 14-17 inches. These numbers can't be guaranteed accurate but will give you an idea of where you stand.

What muscles are you looking to strengthen?

For you to improve your vertical jump, you will need to target the muscle areas that are responsible for propelling you up. Below are some examples of muscle groups that you need to target if you want your vertical jump to go up.

- The Gluts

- The Quads, or thigh muscle

- Hamstrings

- Calf Muscles

- The Ankle Plantar Extensors are the muscles that raise your heels from the ground.

- The Abdominal Muskes

For those who are not familiar with the concept, they may be surprised that the abdominal needs to be strengthened in order to jump higher. However it is vital to have strong core muscles and flex your body during jumps so you can get more air.

Chapter 9: Factors Affecting Vertical Jump

Before you can start training to increase your vertical jump, it's important to determine where your primary focus is. It takes many muscle groups to be able do a vertical jump. If you are only working on one muscle, expect to be able leap more than two feet above the ground.

To increase your vertical leap, you'll need to know what muscles you must train. This will make your training program more efficient and help you see better results sooner. To get you started on your journey towards gaining more air, these are the key aspects you should pay attention to when you are training.

Quad Strength

The quadriceps foemoris, or more commonly known as "quads", refers to the four large muscles at the front your thighs. The quads are extensors of your knee. If you want your vertical jump increase, these are the muscles to strengthen.

Strong quads will help you jump well. You will notice that your hips and knees will bend when you jump. These movements require your quads to do the bulk of the work.

When you can squat approximately one and a-half times your bodyweight, your quads are strong enough for you to propel you several feet above the ground. If you can do more than that, it is a good sign. Because you'll most likely be jumping from one leg to get your feet up, it is a good idea to do as many single leg leg squats with your dominant leg. You can also do them on your other leg to balance them.

Calf Strength

The calves, which are two large muscles (the soleus and the gastrocnemius), can be found at the back portion of your shins. It is located just below your knees. The medial head and lateral heads of your gastrocnemius muscles are what you can see. The soleus is located in front the gastrocnemius. You'll only be able notice them if you've worked your legs hard.

The calves serve two functions: they plantar flex your feet, which causes your toes and body to point down. Because the calves do most of your jumping work, it's only natural that you want to strengthen them.

Calves need to not only be strong but flexible so they can exert enough force on the ground for you to lift your bodyweight. Jump rope is an excellent exercise that can strengthen your calves. It will also increase your cardio endurance. When you can jump rope long enough to lose count of how many times you have done, you will notice a significant improvement in your vertical leap.

Flexibility

You've never seen professional basketball players dunk the basketball with their bodies stiffened and rigid. You can't use all your muscle power effectively if you have no flexibility.

You will notice a wide range of motion in your muscles when you become flexible. This will allow them to contract more and extend further, increasing your power. You will also be able to jump higher if you have more power in your muscles.

Chapter 10: Strengthening Exercises

Now that you are familiar with the muscle groups that make up the vertical jump, you can begin to strengthen them. There are hundreds upon hundreds of exercises and equipments you can use to increase your jumping power. This ebook will only focus on the ones that do not require equipment but are nonetheless effective.

Quad Muscle Exercises

There are many easy exercises that can be done to strengthen your quads.

Leg Raises

1. Keep your right side straight. Make sure your head, legs, and calves align with one another.

2. Your left hand should be in front, with your right arm extended high above your head. Place your hand on the mat. Relax, and then raise your left foot.

3. You can exhale and lift your left knee. It should be raised for at least 2 second. Keep that position for at minimum two seconds. Then slowly lower the leg to the neutral place. Inhale as the leg is lowered.

4. Repeat steps 1 to 3, ten times. Next, roll to the opposite side and repeat.

*Additional tip: Your quads will get stronger as you increase the number of repetitions. You can also hold your leg up slightly longer to continue your quad improvement.

Lunges

You will need to bring a pair shoes.

1. Steer straight up with your feet shoulder-width apart.

2. Move forward with your right foot and place it in front of your right knee. Your

right knee should be bent at 90 degrees. It shouldn't extend beyond the toes.

3. Breathe in and extend your right leg forward.

4. You can exhale when your right foot is lifted back to the beginning position.

5. Repetition steps 1 through 4, but this time, use your left side to lunge forward. You can do 10 repetitions per leg. If your quads are stronger, increase the number.

Squats

You can do this exercise using free weights such as barbells, dumbbells, and so on.), resistance bands, and/or your body weight.

1. Keep your feet together and stand straight. Your hands should always face your side.

2. Your core muscles should be activated. Now, pull your shoulders back and bring your shoulders down. You should keep your

weight on the heels with your head in front and your back relatively straight.

3. Keep inhaling as you lower your body to the floor.

4. When you are back in a standing position, exhale. To start, do three sets of 10 repetitions per set of squats. As you gain strength, you can either add more reps or free weights to your sets.

Calf Muscle Exercises

Calves are the muscles that will be performing the most work when it comes jumping. This is why you need a lot to train them. These are intermediate and basic exercises that you might want to try.

Standing Calf Raises

1. If you are unable to balance on your feet, then you might want to sit straight up and place your hands behind you.

2. Inhale while activating your core muscles. Lift your heels, and then exhale.

3. Keep this position for at least a minute before slowly lowering your body. Do 3 sets with 10 repetitions. If you are looking for more challenge, resistance bands may be helpful.

Calf Raises Over Steps or Calf Blocks

This exercise is similar to a regular Calf Raise, but it's more challenging.

1. Standing on the edge or using a calfblock if you have one is a good idea. It is important that you have either handrails or something that can be hung onto.

2. Depending upon how flexible you feel, lower your heels approximately 2 to 4 inches below the edge.

3. Slowly raise your body until you are at the tips of your toes. Then exhale, as you lift

yourself up. Keep this position for a few seconds.

4. Slowly lower down until your starting position is reached. Inhale while you do this. Do 3 sets of 10 repetitions.

Jumping Rope

Even though I understand that there was no equipment needed earlier, it is important to invest in some jump rope if the goal is to increase your vertical leap. There are many ways to improve your jumprope skills.

- Never land flat on your stomach.

Keep your time on ground as short as you can. You should always bounce on your feet.

Low Pogo Jumps

1. Keep your knees bent at the knees, and keep your feet together.

2. Jump up and fall as fast, like you're jumping rope. Low pogo jumps can be

performed as a warm-up to the rest of your calves exercises. You can also do pogo jumps high; this is where you use only your ankles, calf muscles and jump as high up as possible (three sets of 10-15 repetitions).

Plantar Flexor Muscle Exercises

The muscles of the plantar flexors "flex" the ankles. In other words, they are the ones that push the ground off when you leap in the air. You can increase your jump by strengthening the plantarflexors. This will allow you to land safely and prevent injury.

Towel Curls

This exercise requires only a bath towel. A few weights may be helpful to make it more difficult.

1. You can sit on a couch with your feet flattened on the floor.

2. Spread the towel onto a smooth surface. You can also place some weight on the opposite end.

3. Move your legs straight up and down, then pull the towel's material towards your face.

4. You can either repeat the process as many times as necessary or pick up small objects on the floor with your feet.

Skipping

It is best to run for only a few minutes when you go on a run. Even though you may seem silly when you're running down the road, your plantar fascia muscles are getting a good workout.

Abdominal Exercises

While your core muscles and abdominals are not near your legs, they can be very helpful in improving your vertical leap. Your center of gravity will be thrown higher by your abdominal muscles. This means that your legs and other muscles don't have the burden.

Crunches

1. To reduce strain on your lower spine, lie flat on you back.

2. You can exhale while raising your upper body a few inches off of the ground. Then, activate as many core muscles as possible.

Bicycle Leg Raises

1. You should lie flat on your back, with your hands above your head.

2. As you exhale, slowly lift your left knee. Then, extend your right arm and point your right elbow towards your left side.

3. Inhale and return to your original position. Repeat the exercise with your right leg, left elbow, and next. Three sets of 10-15 repetitions each.

Lying Leg Rakes

1. Place your feet flat on your back. Keep your hands close to your sides. Your legs should be lifted slightly above the floor, and your knees should bend slightly.

2. You can exhale while raising your legs about 30°. While you raise your legs, activate all of your core muscles.

3. Your legs should be lowered slowly back to their original position. You can repeat steps 1 through 3 ten times to make 3 sets.

*Note - Only move your leg. You should not be moving your head as you lift your legs.

After just a few weeks of these exercises, the essential muscles involved in jumping will become strong enough to allow you to notice some improvements.

Next is to learn how jump properly to make the most out of all that power.

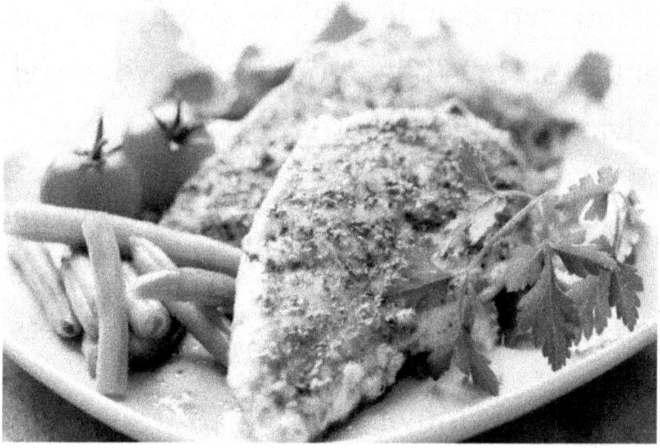

Chapter 11: Improving Your Jumping Skills

As I mentioned in the previous chapter - having enough strength doesn't guarantee that you will have higher vertical jumps. Also, it is essential to master the proper jumping techniques to make the most of your strength. You should also know how to avoid injuries when you jump over fifty inches.

The exercises to improve vertical leaping ability are known as plyometrics. These exercises have been successfully used by professionals trainers and athletes for many years. These plyometric exercises are suitable for both beginners and advanced levels. They will help you improve your strength, as well as teach you proper jumping technique.

Squat Jumps

1. Your feet should be approximately 12 inches apart.

2. To get to the top, you will need to squat so your thighs are parallel with the floor.

3. Start by landing on your feet. Then, jump and squat again. This should be repeated three times, doing ten reps.

Tuck Jumps

1. Start with your feet shoulder width apart. Now, jump as high and fast as you can.

2. While you're still moving up, tuck your knees under your chest.

3. Next, bend your knees and straighten your legs. Land lightly on your feet. Then,

perform a tuck jump. Repeat the process three times and repeat 10 times.

Box Jumps

You don't need a box for this maneuver. Instead, you can use anything between 18 and 24 inches high that's securely attached to the ground.

1. Standing in front of the box with your legs bent slightly and your feet shoulder width apart, place your hands on the floor.

2. Jump onto the box immediately and then jump back down.

3. Jump back on the box as soon as your feet touch the ground.

Depth Jumps

This is basically the opposite from the box jump. First, you need to be on top of the box/bench and then jump down. When your feet touch down on the ground, you can attempt another jump. Continue climbing up on the box, repeating this 10-15 times.

Power Skipping

Skip-skipping isn't just for kids. While it may seem easy and fun, power skipping is hard work.

You will need to perform power skiing by doing a regular skip but adding more explosive energy. Tuck your knee into the chest and you'll be able to skip but take huge leaps.

Lateral Jumps

In addition to jumping forwards and backwards, you should also practice your side to side jumps. Placing a small cone of plastic on the ground should allow you to jump above it. Jump sideways on the other side of a cone. When your feet touch it, jump back. Repeat this process 10 times.

Hurdle Jumps

It is possible that you will need some collapsible hoops for this exercise.

1. You should place the hurdles in a way that they are easy to jump over one after another.

2. Jump over the obstacles with your feet close together. Use your arms to assist.

3. Jump as fast and high as you can over the hurdles. Do this 12 times. Then, jump over the hurdles 3 times with a 1-minute rest in between.

Stair Jumps

1. Place your feet in front a staircase and then jump up onto it. Use double arm swings for support.

2. Once you are on the landing platform, move immediately to the next step. Continue this process until you reach the top.

3. Once you have increased the height and distance of your jumps, you can add steps to each jump.

Vertical jumps

1. With your feet in front, stand straight up and select a point from your ceiling.

2. Jump straight up, and you will reach the destination you chose.

3. If you land immediately, jump up again. Every time you jump, you will be able to reach higher.

You don't need to do them all at once. You can simply mix them in with your normal workouts and still see impressive results.

Chapter 12: Preventing Unwanted Damages

You want to see results immediately, but you also need to be safe when you train. If your body is trained recklessly, you are most likely to get hurt. Then all the gains you have made will be lost.

Here are some helpful tips to ensure that your training is injury-free.

Choose the right shoes

For the majority of the exercises, you will be landing and jumping on the feet. For your feet to be safe, you should wear training shoes that provide adequate arch support.

Wear loose, comfortable clothes

Don't wear clothes too tight. They will restrict your ability to move freely. It's great to have a comfortable shirt, shorts or sweatpants.

Before you start to exercise, be sure to warm up and stretch.

Preparing your body to take the strain you will put on it is essential. Before you do any heavy lifting or other exercises, make sure to stretch your muscles and joints. You should warm up before you start your training.

Make sure you are well hydrated

You will be losing a lot in sweat so it is important to replenish your body's water reserves as often as possible.

Stop immediately if you feel any pain

While some people think it is OK to exercise through pain as it makes you stronger, it is important to be more attentive to what your body is telling you. It is best to stop exercising when you feel extreme pain, especially in your joints. You can consult your doctor to determine the root cause, and the best way to prevent it from happening again.

Don't train too hard

Don't overstrain your muscles or joints by doing too much. Learn to be patient and understand your body's limits. Follow the instructions exactly. You can only increase the difficulty of the exercises once you have become familiar with the previous exercises.

Before starting to exercise again, allow your body to rest.

Do not train every day. You should at the very least, vary which exercises you do. Plyometrics can be very taxing on the body. It is best to give your body a rest before you return to this type of training. Your muscles will not be able to recover from the constant training if they are constantly working hard.

Before performing any of these exercises you should consult your doctor

High-impact exercises can only make your condition worse. If you are considering any type of exercise, including high-impact ones, you should first consult your doctor.

Chapter 13: Why is vertical jumping important?

How do you measure the athleticism of sports? Many would agree that a 40-yard sprint is an indicator. It might be worth considering the weight that someone can lift using a bench press. It is also possible to use body-related metrics.

The percentage of muscle and body fat in an athlete is determined.

Although each measure has its place, the only skill that predicts athletic ability is the vertical jump.

What does the vertical leap tell you?

Professional coaches claim that they can see the athlete's vertical jump and identify his or her explosive power. In basketball, explosive moves are crucial. Players must be quick, strong, and dominant. A coach can use the vertical jump to determine how fast an athlete can move. The vertical leap can also be used to measure the power in an athlete's body.

Athletes might be able use the vertical leap test to see if their workouts are helping them to reach their personal goals. The best way to assess athletic progress is with a vertical jump, according experts. The vertical jump can be performed every other week to help athletes keep track of their progress and adjust their training programs accordingly. Vertical leaps are a great test of athletic performance, as they reveal how explosive and powerful an athlete's body is.

Who should be concerned about the vertical leap

Vertical leap is essential for athletes in all sports. That is why even NFL players have their jumping skills tested at the annual NFL Combine. You can think of the athletic capabilities that are necessary for a wide receiver (or a defensiveback). For football players, leaping is an essential skill. Your ability to jump could mean the difference between a winning play and an intercept.

It is possible to improve your vertical leap for athletes of all disciplines. It is possible to improve your athleticism through practicing and refining your vertical leap. You can achieve success in many athletic pursuits by being able to jump high. Basketball is perhaps the most dependent on vertical jump.

How can a better vertical jump help a basketball team?

Aerial stylings are what made the greatest players of the game. Blake Griffin to Michael Jordan, NBA and college players have all had "ups" that are notable. However, do not let their dedication to jumping fool you. It is not about showmanship. It is.

It is exhilarating watching your favorite player do a dunk on a member.

These opportunities exist in everyday competition, but opposition is rare.

Vertical leap gives you several advantages over your fellow teammates:

* Improved rebounding ability

* Allow extra time for adjustments

* More effective blocking

* Strong shooting ability to defeat defenders

* Showmanship skills for dunking, and other activities

A higher vertical jump will allow you to score more

The fact that vertical jumpers with greater skill levels are more likely than others to contribute more value to a team is undisputed. Not because they are trying to improve their game, but because they can jump higher and have better accuracy.

Advanced players will find the extra fraction of a second in air valuable for tuning a mid-range and three-point shot.

It's common for defenders of the opposing team force players to change their shot's trajectory. The other way it works is that while you may have a certain approach to your jump, a defender might ask you change the direction of the basketball. This decision needs to be made quickly. If you have a high vertical leap you can take extra time to make your decisions.

This ability allows players defeat even the most difficult defenders. This ability increases the likelihood of players scoring points. It doesn't matter if you are looking for that perfect three point shot, or deep in the court, being able outjump a defensive opponent will help you.

Vertical jumping is a key precursor to the obscure concept of hangtime. It seems that top basketball players can stay in the air much longer than less-experienced ones. You can improve this skill only through practice. But, it is essential to develop game-changing hang time skills.

The vertical leap of defense

You might think that vertical leaps are only relevant for offensive plays. Your perspective on vertical jump is limited to scoring points. This is unfortunate. The vertical leap might be more important in some defensive situations. A vertical leap that is higher than the average can help players score more rebounds. Vertical leaps are also useful for defense against shots coming from all directions. Defenders have the ability to prepare for actions deep in paint. They can also stop scoring from mid-range jumpers, as well as the three point range with a dominant horizontal leap.

Although center forwards are taller than the rest of the team, they must still improve their vertical jump. This will enable players at those positions to fight for more rebound. If the vertical jump of a competitor is just an inch higher, it will make it easier for him to get rebounds. Additionally, smaller players can easily overtake players lacking vertical jumps if they are determined to improve their vertical leap.

A higher vertical leap may help improve defensive abilities such as blocking shots and getting a hand in your opponent's face. With a dominant vertical leap, smaller players can become formidable defensive adversaries. Many players are skilled vertical leapers and make great defenders. If you have been told you are too short to play basket basketball, then you can prove them wrong!

This is a demonstration of a great vertical jump.

How to use this guide to improve your vertical leap

This comprehensive guide will give all you need to improve your vertical leap, and make your team a force in basketball. To help you improve your vertical jump, our experts have researched the best diet and exercise programs. You can improve your vertical leap with practice and patience. However, this attribute could be a key to your success in basketball.

Respect for the exercises

Nutritional and other information

The plan includes the following:

Get a better vertical

jump. You too, can dominate

The competition was won

More rebounds and more scoring

You get more points regardless of your age

You can play at any level Don't get left

Behind by coaches simply

Because your vertical leap

You are not up to standard. Follow our

Here are some guidelines for your success

Vertical improvements

Jump up and get started living the

The life you want to live an active lifestyle!

Chapter 14: The Exercises

It is crucial to train your vertical jump in a systematic manner, just as with any strength or exercise program. You won't be able to do all the exercises we provide in this article.

It is important you choose exercises that complement each other and target different muscles. Do not focus on one area of your body in a workout. It can put too much strain on your body, and could cause injury. Your doctor must approve any exercise plan before you can begin. You should always take the time to stretch before you begin, and cool down afterward.

Let's find out what muscles are needed for training and which workouts can help. To begin with, most exercises can be done in two sets. As you move on to the next level of your program, you will need to do three sets.

Hamstrings

The hamstrings can be described as a group of muscles located in the back part of the leg. They are the first muscle to be activated during a jumping sequence. If your hamstrings do not get enough stretch or strength, you won't be able achieve the power that you want. Here are some exercises.

1. Leg curls - Seated

Use a standard kitchen chair. To avoid leaning forward, wrap the arms around the back. Push your heels towards the chair's front legs. Tend the pose for about 10 to 15 second.

2. Body squats

Start by putting your heels shoulder-width apart. Start by extending your arms fully in front, parallel with your shoulders. Slowly sink into a squat. Do not lean forward. You should keep your back straight. Perform 8-10 reps, and then slow down.

3. Lunges

Standing straight up, bring your feet together. Lift your left leg and reach out with your feet together. Now, take a step forward with your left leg and bring it back to the starting position. Do 10 to 12 lunges. Repeat the exercise with the second leg.

4. Power jumping jacks

Start by placing your legs shoulder width apart. Jumping jack. Allow your body to fall into a squat when you land. Slowly sink into your landing, then slowly explode upwards. Do 8 to 10 additional jumping jacks.

The Quadriceps

The quadriceps are the most powerful muscles in your body. They are located just above your knee. Because quadriceps work in conjunction with other muscles like the hamstring or hips in sports, it is important to exercise your entire lower body. Here are some exercises.

1. Box jumping - plyometric

Jumping involves quick muscle movements so it is important to get your muscles working quickly. Get a plyometric kit. These are available in many sizes and heights. A handy exerciser could even make one. Beginners should be able to reach a lower height. Your feet should be about shoulder-width apart. Bring your knees up to 90 degrees, with your arms pointed towards the back. Jump up onto the top box. Reverse the direction of the box and jump off it. Jump backwards once your feet touch the floor. Do 8 to 10 repetitions.

2. Single-leg extensions for single-legged seated positions

These are very similar to the seated leg curls from the section of the hamstrings. However, the leg goes outside, instead of inside. Sit down in a standard kitchen chair. You can keep your arms in front of the chair by wrapping them around it. Place your feet on the flooring. Your left foot should be on the floor. Keep your right leg straight up so it is parallel with the ground. Do 12 to 15. Repeat the process with the second leg.

3. Single leg jumps

Start by placing your feet together. Then, raise your left leg up off the floor with your toes pointed.

backwards. Even if you raise your leg off the ground, your knees should still be straight. Jump five times using your right leg. The jump can be quite small and comfortable. Simply lift your right heel off the ground. While you are jumping, place your hands on the top of your head. Do the same with your left leg. Continue to do this for one minute. This will increase the strength of your quadriceps muscles and your calf muscles.

Calf Muscles

Your calves are located below your knees in the lower part of your legs. They extend down and around the Achilles tendon. Here are some exercises.

* Calf raises

Start with your feet together. Lift your toes up. Do not let your heels touch or contact the ground while you are lowering your heels. Do at least two to three sets with 15 to 20 repetitions.

* X dot jumps

Use athletic tape for marking an X on the surface of your workout. Each point should be between 15 and 20 inches apart. Start at the top left corner of your X. Then jump to its top right. Then, jump to your middle, the backleft and the backright. This completes one cycle. When going back up, go back right, back left, middle, top right, top left. These can either be done on one or two legs. For 30 seconds, start slow and work your way up. See how many you can do.

* Line Jumps

Mark a line measuring approximately one foot in length with athletic tape. Start by placing your feet together along one side. Jump back and forth quickly over the line. See how many you get in 30 seconds.

The Old Standards

These exercises are something you've probably done in gym classes or on the playground. However, don't overlook their value for this program.

1. Jumping rope

Include it in your workouts or do a little bit of jumping rope while watching a sporting event.

2. Hurdles

There are no expensive professional-grade hurdles that you need to overcome. Instead, create your own hurdles using PVC pipe with T-shaped connectors. For spreading on a grassy track or field, four should suffice.

3. Stomach crunches

Another variation of the sit up is to do stomach crunches while lying down. You can use your ab muscles to lift your shoulders up enough to be able to stand on your own. Begin slowly for a minute and then increase your effort.

Each workout should include one exercise.

You should work your quadriceps and hamstrings.

And calf muscles. You can also add some of

The old standards. Start with you

comfort level. Complete a full-cycle

Do the following exercises.

Do the exercises. Work towards doing

Each exercise can be repeated three more times.

You can do your workouts by working out. Don't

You can go overboard to the point where you end up

injury. If you feel pain, stop.

consult your doctor. This will allow you to improve your vertical leap, and your game.

Chapter 15: The Diet

Now that we have covered the muscle groups used to increase your vertical leap, you can probably improve your basketball skills. It is important to work out regularly to improve your vertical leap.

Wrong!

Athletes in all sports

require special nutrition

You can also find diet plans that will help you be healthy.

They receive all the nutrients

Their bodies need.

Basketball is no exception.

different. However, it is.

Recognize this fact

The simple fact that basketball

Players have unique caloric requirements and nutrient needs. They may be different from those of a weightlifter or football player. This chapter contains all the information that you need on hydration as well macronutrients, vitamins, and minerals. This will allow you to take your vertical leap up a notch by balancing all these factors.

Hydration: The building block of performance

Let's face reality: Atheletes sweat. Though sweating is a wonderful way to cool our bodies,

bodies, excessive sweating

Dehydration can occur if you don't get enough water. Remember that dehydration can not only be harmful to your health but also make your performance less efficient. Your heart must work harder to get blood to your major muscles groups. Exercise,

If you aren't properly hydrated, it will make your vertical leap much more difficult.

Scientists have discovered that most NBA players are severely dehydrated before their game begins. Imagine the improvement in stats that would be possible if athletes were properly hydrated. Start the game right and you'll have trouble keeping your hydration in check throughout the contest. A comprehensive hydration plan will help keep your major muscle groups in peak condition, allowing you to retain the explosive power necessary for a great vertical jump.

Before the game

Pre-hydration can be crucial. Two hours before your game begins, ensure that you have at least 16 glasses of water. Continue drinking 8 ounces of water about a quarter-hour before the game starts. Remember, by the time that you feel thirsty you're already dehydrated.

During and after the game

Many of your friends are.

Probability already

Hydrating well

During the match, but

Here are some suggestions:

reminders. You will

Probability of losing between 2 and 4

Drink up to 3 liters sweat daily

Drink up to 3 liters sweat daily

liter soda bottle! That fluid must be replenished. It is important to drink at least 8 ounces per 10 to 20 minute of game play.

After the game

It is now time for you to recover. You should drink 24 ounces of liquid immediately after the game. It does not need to be water.

Basketball experts believe that heavy-protein fluids are extremely beneficial after prolonged exercise. Do you believe chocolate milk can be a suitable choice? That's right! It's a childhood favorite and can help retain the nutrients after a workout. Continue to hydrate throughout your day, even after you've finished the game.

Macronutrients

Now that we have discussed the most important aspect your diet - Hydration - let's get into the macronutrient profile which is best suited for basketball players.

Let's first talk about calories. Basketball's elite players consume between 3,000-4,000 calories per day. You won't need to follow Michael Phelps' 12,000-calorie-per-day diet as a basketball player. Always eat intuitively and "listen to" your body. You won't be led astray by the natural hunger you feel. Maintaining a balanced macronutrient diet is more important than counting calories.

Now let's get back to the macronutrients. Here are these famous macronutrients, in case you're not familiar:

* Carbohydrates

These starchy foods include:

Vegetables, fruits and

sugars. These nutrients

They are crucial for building

How to keep your hair long.

Lasting energy for a

strong vertical leap even

Deep into the game.

Look for complex carbohydrates in brown rice and other unprocessed cereal products.

These include:

* Whole grains

* Fruits

* Veggies

* Rice

* Pasta

* Fat

Energy for

Training long-term

Sessions and support

Get nutrients and absorb them

minerals. Minerals are essential.

You should focus on unsaturated fat.

Because it contains

For components essential

Physical performance

and cardiovascular superiority.

These include:

* Fish (fatty varieties such as salmon)

* Nuts

* Olive oils

* Avocados

* Eggs

* Proteins

A modest amount

protein helps build

muscle. But be careful.

As with all others

macronutrient, if you

Too much protein?

It will be converted

directly into your body fat Protein supplements should not be necessary if you have a balanced diet.

These include:

* Beans, quinoa, and other legumes

* Beef

* Poultry

* Pork

* Nuts

* Hummus

* Soybeans

Experts advise that basketball players should eat about 60% carbohydrates, 25% fat, 15% protein and 25% fiber.

This may be surprising as many exercise routines are heavy on protein. Fact is that athletes need to consume high amounts of calories. To keep their bodies functioning at peak performance, they will need foods with the "sticking power," or carbohydrates. A balanced diet will enable you to maximize your training, and allow for greater vertical leaps.

Vitamins, minerals

Numerous scientific studies prove that athletes need several vitamins. These vitamins include vitamins B and vitamin D. These nutrients are found within the

What you eat on a daily base.

B vitamins are essential for the body to produce energy.

They also promote tissue healing after major workouts such as

weightlifting. Vitamin B12, one of the most essential vitamins, is also important.

The B vitamins. Along with B6, B6 and Folic acid, you can find other vitamins in a variety foods such as:

* Fortified cereals

* Shellfish

* Fatty coldwater fish like salmon

* Skim milk

* Cheese

It may be beneficial to prioritize foods high in B12 and other B vitamins, when you choose your proteins and fats.

Athletes must not only encourage healthy muscles but also maintain healthy bones. This is especially important to those who are involved in jumping or subject their bodies to significant impact. Vitamin D is necessary for the maintenance of bones and skeletal muscle. Vitamin D is important for basketball players who practice outdoors or live in the northern latitudes. Although the sun is a good source of vitamin D, you can also eat certain foods to increase your levels.

These include:

* Tuna

* Salmon

* Portobello mushrooms

* Fortified milk or fortified fruits juices

Recent data shows that vitamins C- and E, long believed to be important, may actually be more potent than we thought.

It is beneficial for athletes

However, performance can actually hamper their muscle

capacity. Because exercise increases the production oxygen, part

A process that builds stronger muscles. Your muscle performance and potential for growth could be at risk if you consume excessive amounts of anti-oxidants such as vitamins C, and E. You should not avoid these vitamins but you should avoid multivitamins with high amounts of them.

The bottom line

Sports professionals are well aware that a balanced diet and special diet will improve athletic performance. A healthy diet will not affect your ability to perform well. If your physician tells you to take a supplement for performance enhancement, please follow their instructions! If you live a healthy lifestyle, and maximize your nutrient levels, you can be a great athlete.

People who want to improve their basketball vertical leap need to train and eat well.

Chapter 16: The Right Support

Basketball shoes are legendary.

Basketball players have always wanted their shoes with a special flair, starting with the Chuck Taylors made of canvas, and ending up with the Air Jordans.

But shoes are much more

Not only does it look good, but it is also very satisfying.

Maximizing results is key.

Your vertical jump. Your footwear

Socks and shoes are essential.

Give the right support

It is possible to improve your leap without injury.

You shouldn't discount socks

Start with your socks. Start with your socks. You should not wear socks. This is because it doesn't protect your Achilles, or the complex network of bones and muscles that make up your foot. It is better to wear socks that you are comfortable with. Uncomfortable footwear should be avoided when you're practicing jumping. Second, you should avoid wearing low-cut socks to improve your ability to jump higher. This will make your Achilles more vulnerable and leave them open to injury. A lot of athletes choose to wear socks that reach their calves and cushioned. Socks made by large athletic-apparel companies are popular because they provide more cushion on the foot's heel. When you leap, your heel is the most vulnerable part of your body. After vertical jumping, the heel is the most sensitive part of your foot. Socks offer extra comfort and cushion to ease the stress of jumping.

There is no single shoe that can help you jump higher than others. Your commitment and hard work will help you jump higher, not the type of shoe you're wearing. You don't have to buy these shoes, even though there are many NBA superstars who have made them available. Choose comfortable, well made high-top shoes, not those that reach your ankles. These shoes may seem lighter and allow you to run faster, but you shouldn't wear them when you are jumping. They are too unstable and provide no support or cushion for jumping. You can cause serious injury to your Achilles tendon, which could lead to permanent physical damage.

There is no single shoe that will make you a better runner or jumper.

It is important to choose shoes that are sturdy and look durable. Shoes are an investment.

It is your investment and you expect it to pay off. Test out several styles of shoes to determine comfort and sturdiness. It is important to choose the best-made shoes. If you want to avoid any potential hazards or distractions while jumping, you should look for the shoes that are the most comfortable. High endurance shoes should have no rips on the sole. This will prevent you from falling hard when jumping. Online reviews can help you get a better idea about the shoe's durability over time.

The extras

Even though it sounds obvious, when you first put on your new shoes, make sure to take care of the lacing. You should not miss any eyelets. Also, make sure you have the same amount of shoelaces both sides. Once they are done, secure them. It is important that your shoe doesn't become loose and fall from your feet while you're jumping. Double-knotting or triple-knotting your shoes will make sure they stay snug and secure. Running in shoes that aren't properly tied can lead to injury. Although injuries from improperly tying shoes can occur, they are totally preventable.

Ankle braces won't improve your vertical jump. Ankle braces can provide support to your ankles. You can expect your ankles to be subjected to heavy wear when you play basketball or improve your vertical leap. You don't have to wear ankle braces if you jump repeatedly in your workout. However, it won't affect your vertical leap or your ability to do so. There are a variety of ankle braces that you can choose from, including one that requires you to tie them. Make sure you secure them if you have to choose one.

Shoes called "strength shoe" are on the market today. Advertisers for this product claim that using strength shoes when jumping directly leads increase in vertical leap. These shoes differ from regular basketball shoes in that they feature a platform at their bottom. Many people believe there is no noticeable difference between training using strength shoes and traditional basketball shoes. But ask your friends about their experiences or look online for reviews.

One last tip.

While it might seem absurd, it is crucial to keep your eyes open for the truth.

Productive and comfortable

vertical-jump training

You will be able to have a cutting session

You should trim your toenails regularly. If

Have a particularly long time

After you cut your toenail, it may fall off.

As you jump, keep rubbing your foot against the toe of your shoe. The nail could not fall off, and instead stay half on and half off. The nail will eventually fall off, resulting in a painful training session.

Here are some tips on choosing the right footwear for jumping. Always wear both your shoes and socks. Wearing less will result in unnecessary stress on the Achilles tendons as well as your ankles. To ensure you have as little pain when you jump, wear socks that provide some cushioning on your heel. No shoe will improve your vertical jump. However, avoid shoes with insufficient support. Basketball shoes can go for hundreds of dollars. However, the price does not necessarily mean that you will get the best results. You should also tie your shoes properly. A pair of ankle braces may be necessary if your ankles have been affected by the jumps. However, not everyone will find them helpful. Make sure to trim your toenails on a regular basis. To prevent you from hindering your ability to increase your vertical leap, don't allow any hangnails to get in the way. You should also think carefully about whether you are going to invest in special shoes for your training. They are not the best option for everyone, and can be a waste of money. They don't fit well, so it is best to choose shoes that feel good and are comfortable while you jump.

Neurological & Biomechanical Influences.

* Muscles tend to bounce back when stretched quickly (e.g. rubber band

* Theoretically, the quicker the eccentric contraction, and the more likely the stretch reaction is activated

* To be truly plyometric, an activity must include a movement followed by an eccentric muscle action.

* Plyometric exercise can increase neuromuscular function, which allows for better control of contracting muscles.

1: MUSCULAR EXPERIENCE

* Muscular power depends on 'how long it takes for strength convert to speed.

* Strength to speed conversion in a short time allows for athletic movements that go beyond the limits of raw strength.

* Therefore, an athlete who can perform the free weight squat with very heavy weights over a long period of time and has strong legs may gain less distance or height from a vertical jump than an athlete who is weaker but can generate less force in a shorter period of times.

* While the maximal force output of a plyometrically trained individual may be lower, and therefore may not be as strong, his training allows him shorten the time necessary to reach his maximum output. This allows him to extract more power from each contraction. This is vital in jump events.

2: MUSCLETENON COMPONENT

* Concentric contractions allow a muscle's movement to be caused by its length. A certain muscle cannot concentrically

contract without a limit on the force it can apply.

* However it can produce more force through elastic storage if the muscle is lengthened and loaded just prior to contraction.

* This effect makes it necessary that the transition time between concentric contractions and eccentric contractions (amortisation phases) is very short. This energy is quickly lost, so the concentric stretch must be performed rapidly.

* This is commonly referred to by the stretch shortening cycling and is one mechanism of plyometrics training. After plyometric exercise, tendon stretches. The quadriceps and thighs can feel tender.

3: NEUROLOGICAL CONTENT

* The neurological component can be found in addition to the elastic-recoil function of the musculotendonous systems.

* Stretch shortening cycles affect the sensory response of muscle spindles as well as golgi¬tendon organs (GTO).

* It is believed that the GTO's excitatory threshold is increased during plyometric exercises, which means they are less likely to send signals to limit muscle tension by sending out signals to limit force-producing units. This allows for greater strength and training capabilities, as well as greater contraction force.

* The muscle spinning is involved in the stretching reflex. It is triggered by rapid muscle lengthening, as well absolute length. The muscle has reached great length at high velocity at the end of rapid eccentric contraction.

* This may trigger a powerful stretch reflex in the muscle spindle, which could increase the power and speed of the subsequent concentric contraction. The amortisation

phase must not exceed a few seconds to allow for a plyometric impact.

* The longer-term neurological component is training muscles to contract quicker and more powerfully by altering firing rates and timings of motor units. Motor units peak during normal contraction in a desynchronized manner until tetany can be reached.

* Plyometric training trains the neurons to contract only with one powerful surge instead of several disorganized ones. It results in a stronger, more powerful contraction that can be used to move a large load (such the body) quickly and effectively.

A summary of the review article Plyometric Training 1996 is provided by Lees & Graham-Smith. It states that the mechanisms of plyometric exercise are the storage and reutilization of elastic energy during stretch-shorten cycles, and the stretch reflex.

They cannot be separated. Plyometric training attempts, in practice, to enhance the effectiveness of both.

* Increased muscle force, increased force development, and enhanced performance are some of the benefits of plyometric exercise training.

* There is strong evidence in the literature that plyometrics training results in adaptation at the level muscle fibre, as well improvements in neuro-muscular functioning. Plyometric training does have one downside, which is the delayed onset and persistence of muscle soreness [DOMS]. This lasts only 5 days and does no harm.

*Plyometrics should not be performed alone. Although plyometric training DOES increase performance, its superiority to other forms of explosive strength training such as weight training and conventional weight training has not been established.

In recent times, I have been combining plyometrics with traditional weight training. COMPLEX TRAINING describes this. This topic will be the subject of a future manual.

SAFETY CONSIDERATIONS...

Due to the potential for injury from plyometrics, individuals should only perform them under supervision. Before you can begin plyometric exercise, you must have the ability to move well and be flexible.

CONDITIONING FOR PLYOMETRICS...

As I've stated before, higher than average forces are applied to the musculoskeletal system in plyometrics exercises. Jumpers need to have a sound foundation of general strength as well as endurance.

Most experts agree that it is important to have a solid grounding in weight training before beginning plyometrics. Before attempting depth jumping, an athlete should be capable of squatting twice their bodyweight. You can also incorporate less intense plyometric exercise into your weight training, to gradually condition your athlete.

Begin with the simplest plyometric drills: skipping, hopping, and bounding.

You should limit your training to more difficult exercises, such as single-leg jumping and depth jumping.

The minimum strength requirement is dependent on where it was obtained and the intensity of the plyometrics.

Chu (1998) recommends that participants are able to do five repetitions in the squat exercise at 60%. You should also strengthen your core (or trunk) strength.

Flexibility is necessary for injury prevention and to maximize the effects of the stretch shortening cycles.

Proprioception plays an important role in balance, coordination, and agility. This is also essential for the safe execution of plyometric activities.

Other safety considerations include the following:

* Age - athletes below 13 years old and athletes who lift less than 1.5 times their bodiesweight should not be allowed to participate. Some authors recommend that children as young as three years old can participate in moderate jumps (low intensity) training. It is important to take care when prescribing training programs for pre-adolescents. Smith, 1975. Because of the immature bone structure of pre-adolescents as well as adolescent kids, it is best to avoid high intensity intensive depth jumps (high intensity) (Smith).

* Surface: Some softness is required. Gymnastics mats can be used, however

grass is acceptable. It is not recommended to use concrete or any other hard surface.

* Bodyweight – Athletes with a body weight of more than 240lbs (109kg), should be careful. Low-intensity exercise should be chosen.

* Technique: Before any plyometric exercise can be started, it is important that participants are properly instructed. They should be well rested with no injury to any of their limbs.

Although plyometrics doesn't pose any danger, repetitions of intense, focused movements can put stress on joints. It is important to take safety precautions when using this exercise method. Many people use low-intensity plyometrics for rehabilitation of injuries.

BRIEF HISTORIZATION OF PLYOMETRICS...

Plyometrics' history dates back to 1960 when Russai, Eastern bloc countries and other nations used novel training techniques for their Olympic athletes. Plyometrics was used in the Soviet bloc countries for many years before 1970. Yuri Verkoshansky [the Godfather'of plyometrics] was the original pioneer. Valeri Borozov [USSR] was the first to win the Olympic 100 metres at Moscow. It was then that the rest of the world realized that 'things had improved'. It is evident that these athletes dominated certain sports in this time period, according to their records. Their training consisted primarily of jumping, foot speed drills (also known as training equipment), stretching, and weight training exercises. This combination allowed them to achieve speed development.

The term pleometric can be described this way: Derived in part from the Greek roots of plethyein which means to increase'.

The purpose of plyometrics, today, is to increase explosive reactions of individuals through muscular contractions and rapid eccentric contractions. This can be achieved using several techniques. The first step is to increase the hip flexibility muscles. They are responsible for lifting the leg. This will increase the frequency with which the leg turns during running and improve the alignment of your body during movement. The result is an athlete who can run faster, has more energy, and has greater explosive power. Core training is crucial. Through the study and research of early exercise science, core training was also developed. Core training refers specifically to the strengthening, development, and training mid-section muscles - the abdominal, oblique, lower back, and oblique. This is also associated with faster development.

Plyometrics, a science that is constantly evolving, continues to be a fascinating field. As we continue seeing athletes achieve new heights .....

OK: Enough about what plyometrics actually are. Let's now look at how it could be integrated into a jumper training program.

As I explained above, I have always been interested in Plyometrics. I have read numerous manuals, books, and articles. Last but not the least, one my favorite articles is by Yuri Verhoshansky [USSR] from 1967. While he is frequently credited with the creation of plyometric exercise, the phenomena that underlie plyometrics - a higher muscle force due to eccentric contractions - has been known for at least 1892.

Plyometric-type exercise has also been a feature in jump training since before the term "plyometrics" was created. It was a term I didn't know about back in the late 1970's when I was doing it.

This is the first article I have ever read about the subject. This article is not complete, it's just an overview of the 1967 Issue 'Legkaya Atletika'.

There are many ways to train plyometrically, but my favorite type is Depth Jumping, which involves using multiple boxes and platforms. I'll explain them all in the manual.

Plyometric Platforms

DEPTH JOUMPING IN THE TRAINING FOR JUMPERS...

Based on work by Yuri Verhoshansky, [USSR]

Depth Jumping (or depth jumping) is a special strength preparation program. It's a method of increasing the nerve muscle system's reactive ability.

Depth jumping involves a takeoff following a jump at depth. It is also called logically depth jumping.

WHY JUMP OVER FOR DEPTH

During takeoff, the exterior muscles fulfill yielding work (the phase of amortization) in the beginning and later ending work phases of active takeoff. BUT FIRST - WHAT IS AMORTIZATION?

All plyometric movements are composed of three phases.

* The pre stretch or eccentric muscle movement is the first phase. Here elastic energy is produced and stored.

* The second stage is the time period between the end the pre-stretch, and the start the concentric muscles action. The 'amortization' phase is a short transition from stretching into contracting. The muscle contractions that follow this phase will be more powerful if it is shorter.

* The actual contraction of muscle is the third phase. This is what the athlete actually wants to do in practice: the powerful jump or throw.

This sequence of three phases is known as the stretching-shortening circle. Actually, plyometrics might also be known as stretch-shortening cycles exercises.

It is easy to show the effect of the stretching cycle by performing two vertical jumps.

* The first vertical jump requires that the jumper bend the knees, hips and ankles. This is called eccentric muscle action or prestretch. The amortization phase will increase by 3-5 seconds.

* On the second jump, the athlete bends their knees and hips at the same time but then jumps straight up. This minimizes the amortization phase, and maximizes elastic energy stored. The second jump will go higher.

It is important to note that the nature of work can make a difference in young athletes as well as older, more experienced athletes.

The older athlete is less flexible in the knee joint and has a faster extension of the leg. His muscles move faster from yielding work into overcoming work, and he develops maximum dynamic strength quicker than the beginner.

The older athlete's nerve-muscle apparatus is more reactive. It's possible to say that his muscles can fulfil an effective function of an 'explosive character' immediately after significant loading. His muscles also have the speed to switch from yielding work to overcoming work.

Analysis of muscle work during exercise [jump type, barbell] by jumpers revealed no means that could have been used to develop reactive ability of motor apparatus.

This is a top quality and increases mainly when the jump is performed with full strength and with full runs. New investigations were needed in order to add effective strength preparation methods to the training arsenal for jumpers. This is when depth jumps became popular.

HOW ARE THESE JUMPS COMPLETED?

Jumping directly from heights of 64 to 110 centimetres is the best way for developing reactive abilities. A quick active take-off right after landing is crucial. An object is held at a predetermined height in order to control it. The athlete should reach his hand with his other hand so that the object can be lowered gradually.

To protect the front portion of your foot, place a thick elastic cover or felt on the area where you want to take off. The angle of the knee joint should not be too steep to soften landings in phase amortization.

Depth jumps come in many forms. In this situation, the jump should be approximately 55 cm deep.

Tiefen jumps are based on the fact that the kinetic energies of the falling body are used for stimulation work of muscles and not loaded. This provides sufficient speed and magnitude during the amortization phase. There is also a subsequent switch in the work of muscles during take-off. Additional loading will increase maximum strength but slow down the muscle's ability to transition between overcoming work and take-off speed. This causes the depth jump to lose its essence.

WHY A HEIGHT OF 64cms OR 110cmS?

The take-off from a certain height can result in a significant improvement in the reaction ability of nerve muscle apparatus.

The first height [64 cm] is the fastest speed in switching muscles from yielding work into overcoming work. The second [110 cm] height corresponds to maximum dynamic strength.

The take-off mechanism is affected by any further height increase for depth jumping. The maximum strength and the middle strength of the take-off mechanism do not change. However, the speed at which the muscles convert from yielding to overpowering work is sharply reduced. Also, the meaning of the exercises is lost.

Athletes who are looking to improve their training effectiveness by using a high-height depth jump are similar to the eccentric who follows the principle. Why take medicine with 15 drops twice per day when it is possible for them to take the whole vial at once?

Beginners and young athletes shouldn't do depth jumping. You will get a lot out of repetitions of jumping in motion and place. Jumping with weights and using barbells will also be beneficial.

It is clear that jumping from depth improves the ability of athletes to utilize their strength potential under pre-determined conditions. They work only when used with speed, strength, and reactive explosive characteristics. It is therefore best to practice them during strength preparations or the preparatory period.

It is important that you realize that depth jumps are physically demanding. You should start training slowly. Jumping 32kg is the best method to prepare for depth jumps. This can be done between jumping exercises and gymnastics benches.

HOW MUCH AND WHEN CAN YOU JUMP?

The amount of jumps required depends on the level of training and experience of the athlete. For athletes who are well prepared, it is sufficient for them to jump twice per week. The maximum number of takeoffs after a depth jump should not exceed 40. The basic version of the jump should be repeated 30 times per week by less skilled athletes. The jumps may be performed in series, 10 times starting at 64cms or 10 times starting at 110cms. Each repetition is repeated twice.

Running exercises, relaxation and series can all be combined. General developmental exercises are recommended, which include strength exercises with moderate loading.

Training sessions that are focused on speed strength preparation should include depth jumping. It is also a good idea to add them to your barbell exercise routines. A second time, depth jumping can be performed during sprinting or jumping sessions. It is important that throwers as well as jumpers do depth jumps three to four days prior the main event training.

Contrary to other strength exercises and frequently barbell exercises that can have a similar effect, depth jumps' effects last for six to eight extra days. To avoid injury, depth jumping should be stopped 10-14 days prior the competition. In general, depth jumps should not exceed 10-14 days before competition.

What types of PLYOMETRIC EXERCISES IS THERE?

There are so many options, it can be difficult to choose from. I choose exercises that match the movement patterns of the events that I coach. You should consider the specificity of the event when you plan your plyometric programming.

Jumping is the most common exercise for the lower body. It can be used to increase the intensity and speed up the plyometrics.

Let's take, for instance:

* Vertical leaping on the spot

* Standing jumps for distance

* Jumping down at a height [depth jumps or drop jumps]

* Hops-and-bounding that involves sideways or horizontal movements

* Jumping on boxes or other obstacles

These can be performed without or with apparatus. The apparatus is used for controlling the activity. Raised box or platform.

HOW MUCH EXERCISES AND REPETITIONS IS THIS?

* Don't do too many repetitions in one session. Since it is a quality session with an emphasis on speed and power, rather than endurance, break the work up into sets that allow for plenty of recovery.

* An experienced athlete performing lower body plyometrics may make between 150-200 contacts during a session. For athletes who are new to plyometrics, it is best to start with 'low to moderate intensity' exercises with about 40 contacts per sessions. There are 12 contacts in 2 sets of 6 bunnyhops.

The force of gravity is used in plyometric exercise by having the jumper take off a box. This can be used to store elastic energy and then instantly release it the other way.

Tellez '97 says that "Plyometrics emphasize on two key components of speed strength: explosive strength (which is the ability for a muscle to contract over a distance without resistance) and starting strength (which is how many muscle fibres can be instantly recruited). You can sprint fast for 40 to 100 metres, and other similar movements with little resistance.

He says that plyometrics' main goal is to help a person jump faster and generate more force in a shorter time. For those who are able to recall, Tom Tellez was a coach to Carl Lewis for a while.

You should match the form, strength, and range to which the event calls for plyometric exercise.

You should always exercise in the right direction. Some plyometric movements, such as those for sprinting, should be directed to the rear, since the leg moves towards the rear. The rate at which the stretch takes place is closely tied to how effective plyometric exercises are. The faster the stretch rate, for example, the greater muscle tension and the stronger concentric contractions in the opposite direction.

Although weight can increase resistance, excessive weight (weighted jackets etc.) could increase strength without having any effect on power. This makes plyometric exercise pointless. Your body provides plenty of resistance. The addition of a lot is unnecessary. If you feel the desire to gain weight, then add 1 to 2% to your body weight.

When possible, perform a plyometric activity at a faster speed than you can produce without assistance. Plyometric exercises should be performed at a speed that results in less down time than sprinting. The muscle will contract faster if it is forced into lengthening at a rapid pace. Also, the closer a muscle is to its contraction, the more violent it will contract.

Jumping from platforms and boxes should be done with care. Avoid stumbling upon the ground after contact. The goal is to get down as quickly as possible. By doing this, you are effectively teaching the nervous system to feel the increased speed. It can replicate this in competition."

It is extremely important.

"Do your best to minimize joint flexion when landing. Too much flexion of the legs during landing increases your time on the floor, absorbs most force and allows very little preloading. When the soles of the feet touch, the knees will be quickly flexed into a normal jumping position. It is a fully footed landing. The heels do not touch the floor.

* All exercises must be performed correctly by the jumper. They require skill, and it is

essential to be able to correctly perform the movements. This is critical.

To help balance, authors suggest that you place your knees on the ground or thumbs up with your elbows and hands in front of your body.

Safety Precautions

Researchers have found that injuries are rare, but it is important to pay attention to the intensity and volume at which sessions are held. Sessions should always be monitored. Accidents can occur due to too many sessions per semaine, too many jumps, poor form, jumping too hard, or using plyometrics in an early age without the proper strength base.

NOTE

Too high platforms for depth jumping can increase injury risk, especially to larger athletes. They also prevent the quick switch from eccentric to conscentric activity. The heights recommended for depth jumps range from 60cm to 80cms.

GUIDELINES REGARDING INTENSITY VOLUME & FREQUENCY...

Intensity..

* Amount of effort

* Can be controlled based on the type of exercise done (DL jumping – less stressful then SL jumping).

* Move from simple activities to more complicated

* Increasing the box height or adding weight externally can increase intensity

Volume

* Total work performed in one session

* The total number of foot contacts made in a single session

* Beginners- 75-100 Foot Contacts/session

* Advanced – 200-250 foot contact/session

Frequency

* Maximum frequency suggested for recovery is between 48 and 72 hours.

Guidelines for Plyometric Training Programmes...

* Sound technical foundation

* Specific to the goals of each athlete

* Quality of work matters more than quantity

* The exercise intensity is a measure of how long it takes to recover from an intense workout.

It is best to finish your normal workout with plyometrics training.

* This exercise should be replicated under partial or complete fatigue

Maximize volume if proper technique isn't demonstrated. Once the maximum volume has been reached, the exercise should be stopped

SOME OF MY PLYOMETRIC BILLS...

There are so countless plyometric tools that you could use. Here are 32 drills that have worked for me. There are many more. Many of them can easily be customized to fit your needs. That's half what makes it so much fun!

You can tailor each exercise to your jumpers based on your age and previous experience. You control the number and height of contacts as well as the recoveries.

It is possible to go wrong if you don't work within the physiological, mechanical and psychological implications of the Plyometric concept.

Each drill is accompanied by my explanation and the procedure.

You are developing the explosive, elastic, reactive strength that is required for all jumpers.

1: SIDEWAYS BOX DIRT

This is an excellent drill to include. One platform is all you need. The jumper will jump up vertically and then sideways. This drill can also be timed for any period of time. You could set it for 30-60 seconds, or even 90 seconds. It is an explosive drill so correct body posture is vital throughout the drill.

Coaching Points

* Keep your head elevated and your shoulders back

* First use the arms. However, the exercise benefits will be greater if the arms are used less frequently.

* Limit contact to the floor to a minimum

* Land on the platform with limited flexion to the back of your knee

* Balance, coordination and coherence are crucial

* Reach maximum height when driving from the floor.

2: ALTERNATE BOUNDING INCLUDING DOUBLE ARMS

This is a difficult drill, so you need to be cautious about how far or how many contacts you make.

With a 1 minute recovery time between each repetition, you could do 3 sets 5 contact. This would give you 15 contacts. I've already stated in this manual that my individual plyometric training unit is limited to 150-175 contact.

Coaching Points

* Starting from either a static or short run-on. You can add some impetus to horizontal velocity by using a double arm action.

* Keep your upper body straight, and face forward while keeping the neck exposed.

* Land on the full foot, and try to use the ankle sweepback - landings immediately become takeoffs, so landings must always be active

* There will be no lateral movement [sideways] and only linear movements ("straight line").

3: ALTERNATE BOUNDING W/ A SINGLE ARROW ACTION

This exercise is exactly the same as the previous one, but this time you will only be using one arm. This skill is not only useful for strengthening your strength but it can also be used as a technical drill. Triple jumpers may use either a single- or double-arm action.

4: ALTERNATING Push OFF

I love this drill. The jumper puts his/her foot flat against the platform. They then drive vertically upwards, trying to land as high on the platform as possible. They then set their foot back on the platform, and they place one foot on it.

It is important to work both legs. Alternate between left and right. It is possible to do five on the left side and five on your right. While you could use arms to drive your body vertically, this might not be possible for all. The emphasis should then be on the legs.

5: DOUBLE FOOTED BOUNDING SURROUNDING A SERIES Of HURDLES

This is double-footed bounding over a hurdle, at a set height that is determined by age and experience.

An experienced jumper may place six to ten hurdles in a row. He might perform five sets of six hurdle bounds [30 contacts] each, with one minute recovery in between each set. For each jumper, adapt accordingly.

Coaching Points

* Standing position: Lower your hips slightly, then drive vertically upwards

* The vertical impulse is not triggered by a forward lean.

* With heels slightly raised, land on your full foot.

* Check that the knee joint is not flexed too much

* Immediately upon landing, DRIVE AWAY FROM THE FLOORING FLOOR

6: COMBINATION BOUNDING - [Double arm]

This drill is exciting and highly rewarding. It's done over a specified distance, determined again by the experience and age of the jumper. The jumper runs on up to 10 m and then BOUNDS dynamically forwards. The jumper must be in a wide, split position during the flight phase.

The double arm jumper action is used. The arms are moved forwards and inverted during the flight phase. Your arms should be in the rear for landing. The arms must be very long and rangy.

Landings/take-offs need to be done quickly and with limited time on ground.

Keep your head elevated and keep your upper torso upright.

A typical session would include:

* 6 x 6, with 90 seconds recovery time between repetitions

7: COMBINATION BOUNDING - [Single Arm]

This exercise is similar to the one mentioned above, but it uses an alternate arm. A triple jump drill that is great. These coaching points are exactly the same as for above.

One session might look like this:

* 6x bounds with a 90-second recovery between repetitions

8: COMBINATION BOUNDING W/ VERTICALJUMP

You could mix and match to make a variety of hops and bounds. The plyometric principles will remain the same.

If you are running on a run-on, you can do 2 hops with the left leg: BOUND. After landing, place both legs together and DRIVE vertically towards the sky. You have combined both vertical and horizontal elements.

It all adds to variety and motivates. You wouldn't like to do the exact same exercises constantly. Some jumpers become bored very quickly. !

9: DEPTHJUMP

My programmes tend to include a lot more box and platform work. It's a personal preference. The jumper is standing at the top of a platform, 60-70 cms. He immediately descends and does not get out. It is vital that the jumper doesn't go out but up.

Make sure you land on your feet with no flexion at your knees and that you use that energy very quickly, in fact, almost immediately.

There are many options for this drill.

* Next, land the vertical jump again. Drive forwards into a standing-long jump

* Return to the standing long jump after landing. Repeat this SLJ two more times (or as many as you want).

10: DEPTH JOUMP TO VERTICAL JAUMP TO A 2nd PLATFORM

Another exercise that is adaptable and can be refined. The jumper must stand immediately on the platform between 60 and 70 cms. After landing, the jumper should immediately drive up onto the second platform.

* He/She could complete 2 sets of 10 and have 1 minute recovery time between sets.

For advancement, there are a variety of platforms [6-10].

NOTE: Never forget to reinforce the principles of plyometric use the energy saved immediately, firm landings with little flexion at the knee joint. Additionally, there should not be forward lean.

11: DEPTH JOUMP TO RIM JAUMP [or any high-placed object]

A great drill to increase vertical impulse. Basketball nets can be used as a target for training in a gymnasium or sports hall. This is the drill. You could do two sets of 5 repetitions each, with a recovery time of 1 minute between each set.

12: DEPTHJUMP OVER a BARRIER

Another drill that is simple to set up. A barrier can be almost anything, including a hurdle or a medicineball. The goal is to simply DRIVE rapidly upwards and past the barrier.

13: DEPTH JOUMP TO A STANDING LOONG JUMP

This is a good drill. I use it a lot. The jumper stands up on the platform and falls to two feet. This time, the jumper has to keep his head up and have limited flexion at the knee joint.

The jumper then drives forwards, upwards, and attempts to get maximum distance from the initial landing. It can sometimes be measured.

It is possible to add a vertical jump right after you land from the standing long leap. Remember that your imagination is the only limitation. Make up your own version of this drill.

* 2 sets (5 each) of depth jumps and a standing long jump

* 2 sets (5 each) adding a vertical jump

14: DOUBLE LEG BOUNDING

Another great drill. You can either limit the number of contacts or do it over a set distance (30 mts).

If you have a distance to go, the progression of a person could be determined by how many double footed steps they can accomplish within this distance.

The goal is to make each bound as long as possible, but I have an alternative where they can ask for height and distance. I assign them a certain number of bounds for this drill.

I expect landing to be a little bit flexible behind the knee, upright torso, and good use. Sometimes, I even ask them for their arms to be isolated, as it can be very difficult. They should 'touch-and-go'.

15: FRONTBOX JUMP

I love the drill and use this drill a lot. My jumpers who are experienced have been able to drive me up to a 90cm platform. An average platform is between 60-60cms.

The jumper should be facing the platform. Lowers your hips slightly, then drives up to the top.

They could do two sets each of 10 with a recovery period of 2 minutes between each set. Remember that quality is more important than quantity.

16: JUMP to BOX

This drill is not too different than the last one, except that the jumper must perform a standing jump to land in an upright and limited knee flexion position before driving up onto the platform's top. It can be at any height you choose.

17: JUMP OUT OF BOX TO GET 'FREEZE'

The jumper needs to descend from a platform and land on the ground as shown above. The jumper is effectively FREEZING the landing. The jumper takes a moment to pause and then repeats the process.

* 2 x 10 reps. Between repetitions, you should have 30 seconds of recovery and then do 3 sets.

18: MOVING SLIT QUAT WITH CYCLE

This drill is very difficult and should be practiced frequently. I tend to give it to my more skilled jumpers who have done plyometrics training for a while.

Jumpers must move forwards for a certain distance or do a set amount of split squats. He then drives into a wide-split position, and at the apex of his flight path swaps his legs dynamically landing in wide-split position on the surface. This is not a drill that's for beginners.

You may do 2 x 30m or 2 x 5, depending on how many times you are doing it.

19: HOPS AROUND PLATFORM

This exercise is extremely useful and helps to improve your jump strength as well as timing, balance, coordination.

The jumper is hobbling up to a raised platform in order to land on it. He alternates his take-off and landing legs. Again. My group is constantly asked to limit knee flexion. The angle must match the angle at which the takeoff leg is when it takes off after a full-approach run. They should not feel too compressed as they step up on the platform.

You might do 10 x hops left/10 x hops right.

20: MULTIPLE BOXTOBOX JUMPS - SINGLE LEG PLACEMENT

Use as many platforms/boxes and as many as possible. The jumper jumps to the first platform on two feet and then drops down to land on one of his legs. He adjusts his take-off to land again on two legs, but always falls on the drop to one leg. The jumper can assist by using his arms in the exercise.

Every coach will find many ways to make the jumper more interesting. It is possible to simply use one leg to jump up and down.

You could use 6 boxes for a typical session.

* 2 x10 x single leg only [L & R] and a walk back recovery prior to the next repetition

21: MULTIPLE BOX BOX TO BOX JUMPS

Similar to the previous exercise except the arms have been separated and all effort is transferred to the lower body. Use as many boxes/platforms available as possible.

The jumper that you see above is just moving from one box into the next. When they land on the floor, I encourage them to check their height immediately. I encourage them to take a longer, extended shape when they reach the ground. This encourages them to extend their legs.

22: SINGLE LEG BOUNDING

A very demanding drill. If done well, it will pay off. It takes patience to master this skill.

A jumper runs dynamically over a given distance, or for a certain number of contacts. It is important to be careful when landing. You need to ensure your landing foot is in a straight, flat line. All landings should be fast and active. To help balance, keep your head up and place your shoulders square.

You might do:

* 2 sets (L & R) of bounds, over 30 metres. Each repetition takes 1 minute.

23: SINGLE LEG DEEPTH JUMP

Another one is the jumper, who hops down onto the floor and drives vertically back up in an attempt to achieve maximum height.

PROGRESSION A very demanding drill. It is crucial to ensure that both legs are working.

24: SINGLE LEG HOPS

An explosive, dynamic exercise. This can also be done on a specific distance or in a group of contacts. All the weight is concentrated on one landing. To maintain balance and coordination, make every effort to reduce flexion at each knee joint. This drill is difficult and not recommended to younger jumpers.

* 3 sets of 6 hops [L & R] with a 90-second recovery between repetitions

25: SINGLE LEG PUSH OFF

A great exercise to improve your vertical impulse. You can start as in the diagram below and then EXTEND your leg on the top of the box upwards, landing on the top with both feet. Retrace your steps and continue.

To make the body appear longer, keep it tall.

* Each leg should be set up with 5 sets, each leg having 20 seconds recovery time between sets

26: SPLIT SQUAT SQUAT TUMP

This is similar to the moving splitsquat except that it's stationary. You want to get as high as you can before landing with your legs crossed.

You will find it very tiring and dynamic. Reduce the repetitions to maintain quality. I recommend this drill to more experienced jumpers.

* 2 sets (5 sets) with 30 seconds between sets.

27: SQUAT Depth JUMP

This is an exercise in which the angle at our knees increases slightly. This will increase the amount of time they spend on the ground so it is important to respond quickly and move vertically upwards and forwards onto the second platform or box.

* 3 sets with 8 repetitions and a recovery time of 3 minutes between sets

28: STANDING Jump OVER A Barrier

Another simple exercise. You can use a large cones, medicine balls, various hurdle height etc. In the diagram above, the jumpers used a traffic cone. They are standing up while driving. You can see the mid-point drop, but the arms are moving up with a little sink in the hips.

It is possible to also travel sideways, backwards and over the cone. Remember to use your imagination.

29: STANDING LONG Jump with Sprite

I like this drill very much and use it often. The jumper does an energetic standing long jump but doesn't sink his hips too much when landing. He jumps tall with his feet slightly apart, but together. After landing, he EXPLODES forwards in order to sprint a predetermined amount of distance. I use 5/10/15 or 20, metres.

* Ten sets of 10. Each set has a 1-minute recovery time between repetitions. If I have 20 metres to cover, I give them 90 seconds to recover.

It's a very demanding exercise.................but rewarding.

30: STANDING TRIPLE JUMP

This drill is very technical and I use it a lot both with my long jumpers and triple jumpers. The jump phase is completed from a stand. I often get them to jump in the sandpit.

Not only does it help develop the technical elements of the triple jump, but it also helps to develop the explosive qualities of the relevant muscle group.

* 1 set of 10 reps. There is a 90-second recovery time between each repetition.

31: STANDING TRIPLE JUMP WITH JUMP-OVER BARRIER

This is Drill 30. All coaching points will be the same, but jumpers must focus on the last phase. Once the jumper has done five or more repetitions, fatigue is a factor. Extra concentration is necessary.

* 1 set of 10 reps. There is a 90 second recovery time between each repetition.

32: STEP CLOSE. JUMP. REACH

Similar to Drill 11 Similar to Drill 11

JUMP HIGHER. WHAT IS IT LIKE?

SKILL

Vertical jumping is one of the most natural athletic movements. Many of the top dunkers around the globe have never read or worked with a coach for vertical jumping. Instead they simply spend their time dunkin' every day. This shows that every training program should have a healthy mix of jumping and exercises that are closely related, in order to maximize your ability to jump high. It is also important to periodically check your technique, as little mistakes over time can result in losing valuable inches.

POWER

Many people mistake power for strength. But power is not the exact same thing. In physics power is defined as the total amount of work completed in a specified time. For the vertical jump, power is defined as being strong but also being able to exert your strength in very short bursts. As an example, let's suppose you can squat

500lbs. However, it takes you only 2 seconds for this strength to "turn over". This kind of strength is useless when it comes to jumping. After your feet have left ground, you only have 0.2 seconds for maximum strength. The most skilled vertical jumpers can generate huge amounts force in a matter of seconds, almost as if they're "bouncing" off a surface. You need to focus on strength and quickness in order increase your power.

QUICKNESS AND STRENGTH

While strength work can be useful in a vertical jumping program, it shouldn't take up the majority of your training. While you can work on your strength, it should not be the only focus of your training. Strength exercises should be done in short bursts. This is done mostly through plyometric exercises, which focus on short ground contact time and quick generation force. Later, we'll be discussing the plyometrics exercises that JHP relies on.

5 WAYS to Increase Your VERTICAL

1. Plyometric Vertical Hop Training

The popularity of plyometric exercise has increased over the years. It is often used as a synonym for vertical jump training. This training style was developed in the Soviet Union as a shock method for training. It is responsible for many of the Russian track and field champions of the 1970s. Fred Wilt (American coach and author) coined this term after he saw the unusual warm up exercises that involved various bounds hops and skips by Soviet athletes prior to competitions. In order to improve your muscle strength, plyometric exercises help you do it in a short time. In order to improve your vertical mobility, you will need to be able activate your strength in the shortest possible time. And plyometrics is the perfect way to learn this skill.

HOW DOES PLYOMETRIC WORKS

One thing that all plyometric exercises share is the use of the so-called stretch-shortening cycling. This complicated way of saying it is that all plyometric activities consist of two phases. During one phase, the muscles involved in the exercise are stretched. However, they contract explosively during the second ("shortening") phase. Let's use DEPTH JOUMP as an illustration.

DEPTH JUMP

Step 1: Take a chair or box and place your arms in a neutral position. The box's height should correspond to your general conditioning. For beginners, it is safer and more comfortable to begin with lower heights in order to avoid injury.

Step 2 - After landing, your quads and calves will be stretched by the downward motion. This is the "stretch" phase, where the athlete tries quick to stop the down motion and minimize the time on the ground.

Step 3 - You have reached the lowest point. Your muscles are now stretched to the maximum. Similar to a stretched rubberband, your muscles and tendons have energy that is ready for the next phase.

Step 4: In this "shortening stage", the muscles contract at a rapid rate. This is accomplished by two main drivers. - The conscious energy of the muscles (calves/quads, glutes/lower back etc.).

You can visualize the power of this stretch-shortening process by comparing the heights of two jumps.

1. Deep Squat Jump. Jump from deep squat. This means that your arms must stay straight down, and your knees should not bend at the beginning. Be sure to start your jump at the lowest possible point. Only then, move upwards.

2. Countermovement Jump - You begin by standing straight up and then slowly

descend into the jump. You can bend your knees quickly to gain momentum.

WHAT YOU WILL NOTICE

The countermovement jumping uses the first phase to rapidly descend, much like the depth jump. However, instead of falling from a box, the athletes drop from an upright position.

The athlete can use the stretch shortening cycle to gain speed during the second phase. A deep squat is an unnatural method of jumping. It eliminates the first and thus the stretch-shortening cycles completely. You will find that you can jump higher by using a countermovement in your beginning.

5 Reasons to Do Plyometrics

1. Plyometric exercises can be closely related to vertical jumping so they are a better way to learn the "skills" than pure strength training.

2. Plyometrics is a way for the brain to quickly fire the muscles, which can lead to fast and significant training results. This allows you to learn quickly.

3. Easy to learn and lower risk of injury than heavy lifting.

4. Plyometric Exercises of high intensity also help to strengthen your muscles.

5. Without expensive equipment, you can do exercises to increase bodyweight.

Okay, now you're familiar with the mechanics of plyometrics and why they work so well, let us introduce some of our favourite plyometric drills:

POPULAR PLYOMETRIC EXERCISES TO BASKETBALL PLAYERS

In the following paragraphs we will show eight plyometric exercise options. These can range from simple exercises for beginners to more challenging movements that require strength and coordination. These exercises will improve your vertical jump and increase your ability to jump higher after just a few weeks.

TWO-FOOT ANKLE BOOT HOPS

Standing shoulder-width apart with your feet together, hop continually using only your ankles. You must ensure your knees don't touch the ground and that your ankles extend to the maximum extent possible during each jump. Try to minimize ground contact time. This is an excellent exercise to increase your speed.

SLALOMJUMPS

This exercise is also known "line jumps" since you draw a straight line on the ground. Then, hop as fast and as smoothly as possible. It is important to keep your core stable, look for quick ground contacts and not worry about jumping height. Each hop counts for a repetition. This exercise can be done in the same position or slightly ahead.

POWER SKIPPING

Power skipping can be a great exercise that trains the explosiveness of one leg. The idea is to simultaneously jump high on both the off-legs and keep moving forward slowly. Focus on driving the offleg's knee to the chest while performing the exercise. This will increase your power in your leg swing and your one leg vertical.

RIM JUMPS

Position yourself against a wall, and use your hands to reach the highest place possible.

Jump immediately after landing and then try to touch the exact same point again.

You should be focusing on minimal time on the ground. If the jumps get lower, you should stop.

LEAP FOG JUMP

Begin by standing with your feet about shoulder width apart. Begin by standing with your feet at shoulder width. Now, lower into a 3/4 squat position and extend your arms. Next, try to land on both your toes. Then immediately get up again to do another.

TUCK JOUMPS

Start standing and do a standing leap as high up as you can. Then, lower your knees to the top.

Do not force yourself into a squat.

DROP and FREEZE

You should step off a box between 18-24 inches high. Try to land on both your feet simultaneously while keeping your knees bent.

This is a great exercise to do for weaker athletes, who may not be used to high-impact exercises. This exercise prepares the body to coordinate the high forces during landing, as well as prepares them in depth jumps.

SINGLE LEG DEPTH JUMPS

Single leg jumps are only for experienced athletes. It is important to choose the right height box. The athlete drops from the box as in a regular depth jump, but only lands on one leg. The athlete then tries to accelerate back up as quickly and efficiently as possible. Be sure your knee doesn't buckle, and the center of gravity stays above the jumping leg. For an extra challenge, consider adding a higher box that you can jump onto.

2. Strength Training will help you get higher

Many athletes are obsessed with how much weight they can squat. There's something satisfying about lifting hundreds of pounds on your back. Many people believe that increasing your squat will make you jump higher. You can see that the average powerlifter doesn't believe this. These athletes may be unbelievably strong, but they lack the explosiveness to make a great vertical.

A heavy squat means that you can move a lot more weight very slowly. However the vertical leap is an extremely fast athletic movement so maximum strength is only partially useful.

Strength training alone won't help you jump higher.

It's good news! You don't have to join a gym. It doesn't mean strength training is ineffective. You can use strength workouts with more specific and explosive exercises to really speed up your vertical jump training.

We have one suggestion: Do not begin your training with 40' deep jumps if it is not possible to deal with the intense impact from exercises such as this. But if you feel weak in strength, it may make sense to start your training building a strong foundation.

The following paragraphs contain classic weightlifting exercises, such as the squat which works on maximum strength, dynamic strength exercises that include elements like vertical jumping like Olympic weightlifting, and body weight exercises that you can do without going to a gym.

BODYWEIGHT EXERCISES IN STABILITY

Strong cores are vital for vertical jumping because they provide stability that allows the optimal transmission of force to the upper body from the lower. A weak core can cause you to lose valuable inches during takeoff.

Also, poor posture and lower back pain are often linked to a weak core. These exercises will help strengthen your core.

HIP TRUST

This exercise is great to work the glutes, which is an underdeveloped muscle group in many athletes. Then, place your upper back against a chair or bench and then bring your knees back until your knees form a 90-degree angle. Now push your hips upwards, extending your hips as far as possible. Make sure you squeeze your glutes while doing this move. Keep it up for at minimum 2 seconds.

PLANK

These planks do a great job strengthening your front and sides. It is important to keep your body straight and support your weight with your elbows. You should hold the position for as long time as possible. If you feel strong enough to hold the position for 60 seconds, you can put weights on top of your back to increase difficulty.

RUSSIAN RUSSIAN TIGER

Russian twists are great to strengthen your lower back and oblique muscles. Start with your knees bent. Your back should be at a 45-degree angle to your floor. Hold your arms straight forward and ensure your back is straight. Twist your torso left and right. This exercise can be made more challenging by elevating your feet above the ground. To add an additional challenge to this routine, you can add a dumbbell and/or a medicine bell.

SUPERMANS

This exercise will strengthen your lower back. Keep your arms and legs extended and flat on the ground. Move your arms and legs 4-5" above the floor. Now focus on contracting your lower back muscles. For 4-5 seconds, hold the position. Next, lower your arms and legs to continue the movement.

BODYWEIGHT EXERCISES IN LOWER BODY STREENGTH

Quadriceps muscles and glutes produce the greatest force when a vertical jump is performed. The quadriceps and glutes are the most important muscle groups for strength training. Other muscles, like the calves, spine erectors and arms, have support roles but are often strong enough for jump-specific exercise. The following bodyweight exercises can be used by athletes who don't have weightlifting equipment or access to a gym.

coach. It is not an easy task to do pistol squats.

BULGARIAN SPLIT SQUATS

Bulgarian Split squats target your quadriceps (quadriceps), glutes, and inner thigh. With your front foot flat on ground and your rear foot on a platform, stand straight up. You will now slowly lower into a deep, squat posture. However, make sure your knees are not in front of you toes. For balance, use your back leg but don't weight it too heavily. Move your front foot away from the bench so that you shift the stress to your quads and glutes.

SINGLE EG DEADLIFT

The single leg deadlift, which is great for your posterior chain, is an excellent exercise that will not only increase your strength but also your balance and flexibility. Your foot should be planted on the ground. Keep your back leg straight and your hips back. Do not turn your back and keep your knees bent. The single leg deadlift works well for your posterior chain. This exercise not only increases strength, but also helps you balance and improves flexibility. Your foot should be planted on the ground. Keep your back leg straight and your hips back. You should not round your back and keep your knees straight.

PISTOL QUAT

The pistol sit is undoubtedly the most important of all bodyweight leg exercises. You will need to be strong, flexible, and able to balance in order to perform a smooth pistol squat. It is possible to use assisted forms of this movement. If you find yourself falling onto your back every time you bend too far, it is likely that you lack ankle mobility. You can improve the range of motion at your ankles by stretching your ankle.

EXERCISES TO MAXIMUM TRUTH IN HEAVY WEIGHTLIFTING

These exercises increase your body's maximum power. These exercises are great for any vertical jumping program. However, you should also learn how to use your strength explosively through plyometrics as well as faster weightlifting. As the season begins, athletes will tend to focus on building up maximum strength in the offseason before moving onto more sport-specific and explosive exercises. These exercises can cause injury if done incorrectly so make sure you do them correctly!

SQUATS

There are many different variations to squats. Box Squats can be box squats. Full Squats can also be used. Different varieties place more emphasis upon the quads than others. Others put more stress onto the glutes. As injuries from the squat are possible, make sure you maintain good form. If your back is sloppy or you are having trouble keeping it straight, front squats may be a good option.

DEADLIFTS

Deadlifts will work nearly all the muscles needed to do a vertical jump. They also help activate the hamstrings as well as the spinal erectors. Because it is more natural, trap bar deadlifts are much easier for most athletes. To ensure a neutral spine, lift the barbell from the ground from an elevated position. Sumo deadlifts are a way to lower your body and position your legs wider.

WEIGHTED EXPLOSIVEEXERCISES

Olympic weightlifting, which is explosive weightlifting, can bridge the gap between slow strength exercises that are slower and the explosive and powerful movements associated with a vertical jump. They teach the body how to generate a lot of force quickly and are easy to translate because they have similar movements. You should have a strong core to perform these exercises. When you do these exercises correctly, you can teach your body to use your muscles.

More explosive strength

JUMP SQUAT

This exercise is great to use for vertical jump training. It teaches you how to generate very high power outputs while jumping. It is important to be quick in this exercise. Therefore, only use light weights. The most common mistake is to use too heavy weights. You will lose speed and place too much pressure on your joints. You can also do this exercise without a barbell by holding a medicineball or wearing a weight-vest.

HANG CLEAN

The Olympic lift is simplified and the hang clean focuses more on explosive hip extension. The technique isn't as complex as the other Olympic weightlifting exercise. Vertical jumps can be increased with isolated hang clean workouts.

You can do isolated squat exercises which are probably because it is faster and more powerful than slower squats.

BACKWARD MEDICAL BALL THROWS

This exercise works much the same as the hang cleans but it is much simpler. To throw the ball, hold it between your legs and squat. Keep your legs extended, hips open, and knees bent. This exercise works on your lower body strength and also strengthens your upper body. Your vertical can be as high as 20% with the arm swing.

3. Improve Your Vertical Jump Technique

Vertical jump training should include lots of practicing your preferred jumping style in order to teach the central nerve system how to perform the movement in the best way. Improved vertical jump technique will most likely lead to early improvements in vertical leap height. This is less due to increased strength and power. The best technique for all athletic movements is the one that is optimal. Vertical jumping is a different technique. Most noticeable difference is that some athletes prefer jumping off one foot, while others prefer taking off from two feet. There is no one right way to jump higher, so athletes will pick the type that suits their body best. These are the best techniques for athletes.

ONE-FOOT PLAN

This style is distinguished by short ground contact time, low knee bend and rapid movement of the hips. It requires some coordination. However, proper training can improve even the most natural two-foot jumpers.

TWO-FEET TECHNIQUE

Strong athletes with similar physiques to footballers prefer two-foot jumps. This style features a slower ground contact time and deeper bending of one's knee. Two-foot jumping favors athletes with strong quads and can produce high force in their quads. Athletes who aren't as quick or stiff can still jump impressive heights using the slower two feet jump technique.

4. Better Warm-Ups & Stretching

Vertical Jumping can be very challenging and puts a lot stress on your muscles and tendons. Before starting high-intensity training it is crucial to properly warm-up. This will not only improve performance, but also decrease the chance of injury.

WARM-UP

It is important to warm up before you begin. This will increase your blood flow and raise your heart rate. You could dribble around the court, ride on a bike, or run on an exercise machine. Skipping Rope is an excellent warmup for vertical jump training. It strengthens your entire body, particularly those involved in the vertical jump. You can then move on to the specific warmup after the general warmup of 8-10 minutes. This is the part of the warmup that activates the central nervous system to prepare the body for specific movements. Jump training requires specific warm up exercises.

You could do power skipping or tuck jumps. You can prepare for any lower body strength training session by doing squat jumps, box squats, or power skipping.

PRELIMINARY STRAINTCHING

Dynamic stretching, which allows you make controlled movements and momentum of the limbs and core, is the best practice before a workout. This type of stretching aims to move joints as far as possible, but not beyond their limit. The movements will be relatively short and gradually get wider as muscles and soft tissues cover more joints.

grades.

Benefits of dynamic stretching

- The ability produce more explosive force by using the most elastic muscles.

- Increased blood flow to the muscles and temperature to prepare them for later movements.

- Reducing the likelihood of muscles being torn or stretched.

- A wider range of muscle action which can indirectly benefit weight loss and lean tissue growth.

EXERCISES IN DYNAMIC STRENGTHING

Start by standing straight up. Move forward with one foot so that your leg reaches a 90° angle. Turn your upper body toward the right. Keep moving your left foot forward, bringing it closer to the ground. Continue to twist. End the set by switching sides.

- Start out standing on your left leg, right leg crossed over your left leg. The right foot is the only one that touches the floor. However, it does not have to be weighted. Lift your toes up and lift the leg towards the side. You should keep your spine straight, and your abs engaged. Your left hand can be placed on the wall, or on a chair to help you balance. You can raise your leg as high and low as you want, then place it on your left foot. Do this 15 more times before switching sides.

Stand tall and relax your legs. Now, extend your right arm straight up to your left side. Keep going down until your other foot is covered.

Start by standing straight up, with your hands on your hips. Now, you can rotate in a circular fashion. Turn first to the left, then turn right.

- Start by laying on your back in a plank, your hands on your stomach and your arms under your shoulders. Place your heels behind your head and raise your knees. Engage your glutes, tighten your legs, and brace your core for rigidity. Your feet should be approximately equal width between your hips and your shoulders. This is your starting point. Continue to keep your core engaged as you slowly move your fingers forward. Keep your spine straight and your hips parallel to the floor. You can move your hands as far away as you want, but keep your form. Then, bring them back to the starting position.

STATIC STRENGTHING AFTER TRAINING

Static stretching allows your muscles to be more flexible and allows them return to their natural position. Static stretching should be performed at the end of training after keeping your legs raised for at least ten minutes.

Each position must be held between 30-60 seconds. If the tension builds up before 30 seconds, the exercise will not be sustainable. In the same way, if you are able to hold a position longer than 60 seconds it indicates that there is not sufficient tension to improve any aspect of your life.

STATTIC STRETCHING EXERCISES

EXERCISES OF ADDUCTORS FOR MUSCLES

- Stand straight up with your feet slightly wider that your hip width. Toes facing in front. One step forward, lean your head on the floor and bend forward. Next, stretch one leg forward while keeping the other straight.